Clinical Research Coordinator Handbook

Fourth Edition

Deborrah Norris

Plexus Publishing, Inc.

Medford, New Jersey

Third Printing, 2015

Clinical Research Coordinator Handbook, Fourth Edition

Copyright © 2009 Deborrah Norris

Library of Congress Cataloging-in-Publication Data

Norris, Deborrah.
   Clinical research coordinator handbook / Deborrah Norris.-- 4th ed.
      p. ; cm.
   Includes bibliographical references.
   ISBN 978-0-937548-70-7
   1. Clinical trials--United States--Handbooks, manuals, etc. I. Title.
   [DNLM: 1. Clinical Trials as Topic--standards--United States--Handbooks.
2. Clinical Trials as Topic--methods--United States--Handbooks. 3. Records
as Topic--standards--United States--Handbooks. 4. Research
Design--standards--United States--Handbooks. QV 39 N854c 2009]

   R853.C55N67 2009
   610.72--dc22

                                        2009030187

President and CEO: Thomas H. Hogan, Sr.
Editor-in-Chief and Publisher: John B. Bryans
Managing Editor: Amy M. Reeve
VP Graphics and Production: M. Heide Dengler
Illustrations: David Wetzel, Susan Gray, Bob Jackson,
            and David Beverage Graphic Design
Sales Manager: Linda Chamberlain

Dedication

To Kristen, Nicole, Alex and Baby Jayde, to the constantly amazing life, full of surprises, in front of you and its endless possibilities! Never be afraid to follow your heart or your dreams. Thank you for the love and the joy you bring to my life on a daily basis.

Contents

Acknowledgments

I have watched the amazing evolution and the professional development of clinical research coordinators (CRCs) over the past 24 years.

While CRCs have more responsibilities today (including a working knowledge of the regulations required for clinical trials) and are delegated more tasks, their commitment (first to the safety of their study subjects as well as their commitment to their project) remains. Yet, they still remain unrecognized as the heart of research. While it is not often acknowledged verbally, it is without a doubt known, especially by the clinical research associates (monitors), that there can never be a successful clinical trial without coordinators who care, not only for the quality of their work, following the Federal, State, Good Clinical Practice, and International Conference on Harmonisation guidelines, but first and foremost for their study subjects. It has been an honor to meet and work with these effective CRCs. You are truly amazing!

When the first edition of the *Clinical Research Coordinator Handbook* was printed, I never imagined that there would be other editions or that the first edition would be translated and published in Japan. Throughout this process, over the years, the support and encouragement of those assisting with this edition, as well as the others, have been phenomenal. They have been gracious sharing their wisdom and knowledge, taking the time from their busy schedules to answer my seemingly never-ending questions with patience and understanding, no matter how many times the same question is asked!

It is with continued sincere appreciation and gratefulness that I acknowledge the assistance of many outstanding people in the fourth edition of this handbook.

John Bryans, your continued support from the beginning of our professional relationship to the present has inspired me in so many ways. The professional friendship we've developed over these 10 years has meant a lot. I am honored to be an author with the Plexus Publishing family. Your continued patience and support is one of the reasons there's a fourth edition! Pat Palatucci, I wish you the best of luck in your new endeavors. I miss you.

Thank you to the wonderful people at Plexus Publishing for continuing to believe not only in this book, but in my abilities to communicate with CRCs. Somehow, thank you never seems to be enough.

Thank you to Amy Reeve, a superb editor. Your patience (seems I use that word a lot) and guidance has truly been appreciated. Thank you for understanding a busy pharmaceutical professional has so many study deadlines to meet. It seems the one thing you really want to accomplish is the one thing there seems to be no time to complete.

Thank you to everyone who has reviewed this edition of the handbook, not only for their comments and suggestions but for their belief in this book. This kind of support and encouragement is rare. Your input has not only been invaluable but instrumental in the development of this edition.

John Wilkes, your insight, suggestions, and review of the content have been invaluable. Thank you for being a second set of eyes and my sounding board for just about everything! John, you were my first friend when I moved to Florida; those days teaching at Ward Stone College seem like a long, long time ago. I know we have both enjoyed seeing the students we taught working as medical assistants and in, some cases, CRCs. Sean Kennedy, thank you for sharing your information about electronic data capture. Your friendship and incredibly positive outlook on life is contagious. Thank you for being there in the good times and the bad times, for always seeing the glass as being half full not half empty. You have encouraged me in more ways than you will ever know. J. D. Davidson, once again, thank you for writing the foreword for every edition of this handbook and for taking the time from your busy schedule to assist with the editing of this edition. You knew me when … I value our continued friendship over the past 25+ years. Who knew? Karen White, Maureen Muier, James Mathney, and Brian Dischler, thank you for assisting in the review of this handbook; your suggestions and comments were right on target.

Peggy Miniter, working with you has been challenging and rewarding. I am grateful to have had the opportunity to work with your team. I can never thank you enough for your calls over the past summer; they were not only helpful—your calls showed the level of your managerial support for those working on your team. Thank you so much for your kindness. Tim Carter, I wish you the best of luck in your new endeavor. I will miss your encouragement, support, and advice. I have been fortunate to have had you as my CMS manager. I know it has been challenging at times. Dr. Kevin Cleveland, Dr. James Calandruccio, Dr. Mario Werbin, and Dr. Richard Levine, it is comforting to know, first hand, that there are medical professionals willing to go the extra mile to ensure the best medical care possible for their patients. It is rare to find such caring, competent physicians. Thank you, not only from me but from all of your patients! Deena, my dear friend, you are an amazing woman! Thank you for keeping me focused when I am going in 10 different ways at the same time. Charlie is a lucky man! It is hard to believe almost two years ago we were in Europe. It truly was a "trip to remember," from the flight to Rome to the cruise home. It really was a life-altering experience. To think I never knew fish could fly! Jim, Irv, and Lonnie, from, as Irv would say, "my memorable entrance into the ship's dining room the first night," to our continued friendship, and visiting you, Lonnie and Jim in Salt Lake City, Utah. Jim, you throw unique parties! You are all great guys—wonderful dinner companions—and a lot of fun to be around. Thank you all for confirming my belief there are things that do happen for a reason! Father James A. Quinn, you have helped me in ways you will never know. Your continued encouragement and your belief in my abilities mean a lot to me. Regardless of the need or the reason, you have always been there for me. You and St. Matthew will always have a special place in my heart. As you would say, "Thank you, thank you, thank you."

Nicole, I will never forget your kindness and care when I needed it most. To think the first professional basketball game you ever attended was with the last person you thought loved basketball—

your aunt! You are a great student, great mother, and even greater niece. You will make a great pharmacist. I am so proud to be your aunt. Kristen, watching you grow into a beautiful, intelligent, kind woman has been a joy. There are things in life that happen for a reason, and learning to deal with these surprises is what life is all about! Remember, you have the ability to do anything your heart desires, and yes, you can reach for the stars! Aunt Jeannette and Uncle Roswell, I miss you both so much. Our memories will be cherished for as long as I live. Aunt Jeannette, Rexine has been good to me, too. Marino and Lavinia Robins, there are no words that can ever express my gratitude for your kindness. There are some seeds that take root, but are slow to bloom, and I believe with all my heart the seeds you both planted will grow into giant redwood trees!

Maylee Wong, from the first time I met you (you were just 14 years old) I knew you would continue to grow as beautiful inside as you are on the outside (and for those of us that know you, that says a lot!); you are a confident, wise, loving young woman. Baby Jayde has an amazing mother. Justin, continue to do the right things for the right reasons. Take those lessons you have learned and use them as motivators while you continue your life's journey. Someone once said, "It is not the story that matters, it is the results that count." Remember you are limited only by your mind. Embrace life with its constant surprises and wonders with hope, integrity, honesty, generosity, and kindness so that anyone passing through your life becomes a better person for having known you. You are a good, kind man. Justin, you continue to make me proud to be your mother.

Once again, for technical expertise about the legal portions of this handbook, I went to my ultimate informed source, sounding board, and personal counsel, Francis X. Sexton, Jr., Esq. Any errors or oversights are mine. Allan Silverberg, David Wetzel, Bob Jackson, and Susan Gray, your illustrations continue to bring these chapters to life, while adding some humor. While things continue to change drastically in the pharmaceutical industry, the CRC's role has become even more pivotal to the success of any clinical trial.

To all clinical research coordinators, you are, and will continue to remain, the *heart* of research! I hope the information in this handbook will continue to assist you in your clinical trials.

Foreword

In this short book, you will find a straightforward explanation of clinical research and the role of the coordinator in such research. You will learn that, by following the details, paying attention to them, and maintaining an attitude of strict integrity, you can accomplish a creditable clinical research project.

Deborrah Norris has been doing clinical research longer than she will want me to admit. I have known her from her days as a college student, where she further honed her writing skills as a composition student. She has always been a diligent worker who manages details very well. A strong work ethic and innate sense of integrity have been hallmarks of her work. A candid way of getting to the root of issues is manifested in this handbook. The humor throughout furnishes a welcome segue for the presentation.

Welcome to the world of clinical research!

J. D. Davidson, Professor
Utah Valley University
Orem, UT

I. Introduction

The purpose of this handbook is to outline the various functions required of the clinical research coordinator (CRC), research nurse, research assistant, data coordinator, or medical assistant involved in the conduct of a clinical study for an Investigator on behalf of a pharmaceutical company or device manufacturer and contract research organization (CRO)/site management organization (SMO), which is the Sponsor or Specialty Research Network.

The complete and accurate accumulation of information specified in the study Protocol and the subsequent accurate transfer of this information to the case report form (CRF) or via electronic data capture (EDC) is vital to the successful progress of a clinical study. As coordinators of this operation, CRCs continue to play an integral role, often without the recognition and credibility they deserve for their dedication to this process. This handbook describes the various duties of CRCs and those assisting in the conduct of a clinical study. It outlines the national and international regulatory requirements that must be followed when conducting a clinical study. The documentation that is required before the conduct of a study is described and templates of forms, checklists, and letters are included as tools to assist you in performing your tasks. In addition, the topic of legal liability as it relates directly to the CRC has also been incorporated. There is a new chapter regarding EDC as it relates to the responsibilities of the CRC. An expanded glossary of terms is located at the back of this handbook to aid in the understanding of the language of clinical research. Information regarding patient record privacy (HIPAA) regulations is also included.

Ultimately, it is the close communication, which is essential, between the Investigator, CRC, and the Sponsor that will ensure the timely and successful completion of the clinical study. Studies performed in accordance with their approved Protocol, with the guidance of the Sponsor, and under the supervision of a well-informed, experienced clinical research associate (CRA), will meet the goals of Good Clinical Practice (GCP) and International Conference on Harmonisation (ICH) guidelines, as well as the Federal Regulations established by the Food and Drug Administration (FDA).

This handbook is written as an introduction for the CRC who has not previously been involved in extensive clinical trials, for the CRC who has limited experience in the conduct of clinical trials, and as a refresher for the experienced CRC. There is also information for the Principal Investigator (PI), who is ultimately responsible for assuring that the conduct of the clinical trial is in accordance with legal regulations. In all cases, we are confident that the reader, regardless of his/her level of experience, will gain a more detailed appreciation of the clinical study process.

II. Federal Regulations Governing the Obligations of Clinical Investigators of Regulated Articles

A clinical study is an experiment that has been designed to prove a hypothesis: for example, that Drug A is as safe and effective as Drug B; that a drug's pharmacokinetics remain unchanged in subjects with renal insufficiency; or that concomitant administration of an antacid with the drug has no effect on its absorption or other kinetic parameters. As with any other scientific endeavor, the conduct of a clinical study demands that good scientific methods be rigorously adhered to in order to ensure the highest quality results. Over the past several decades, clinical researchers have developed standard methods that, when implemented in a clinical study, contribute to its smooth progress. These methods may include the use of recog-

nized screening criteria for assessing subject eligibility, such as the use of the DSM-IV to categorize mental illnesses or the use of American Rheumatology Association criteria for determining the extent of involvement in subjects with rheumatoid arthritis. Other elements that add to the strength of the study include adherence to a well-defined clinical Protocol, the selection of appropriate tests to assess safety and efficacy, the use of well-designed case report forms (CRFs) to ensure unbiased data collection, and the use of appropriately applied statistical tests for the analysis of the data.

Collectively, these elements form the basis for the concept of Good Clinical Practice (GCP) and International Conference on Harmonisation (ICH) guidelines. GCP guidelines have been promulgated by the Food and Drug Administration (FDA) with input from researchers, statisticians, clinical personnel, regulatory and legal specialists, and the pharmaceutical industry. They provide guidelines for essentially all aspects of conducting a well-designed and well-controlled clinical study. While it is the Sponsor's responsibility to ensure that a study conforms to the guidelines set forth, the CRC and Investigator also have some legal responsibilities in adhering to these guidelines.

The regulations and guidelines of ICH and GCP are detailed, and the reader should recognize that the elements described in this manual are rooted in these concepts. The Code of Federal Regulations (CFR) 21CFR Part 50, "Protection of Human Subjects," and 21CFR312.50, Subpart D, "Responsibilities of Sponsors and Investigators," describe in detail the regulations set forth by the FDA regarding the testing of drugs in humans. Further FDA-related helpful sources, including online courses, certifications, etc., can be found in Appendix I, Part B.

III. The Clinical Research Organization

A large portion of clinical studies sponsored by the pharmaceutical industry are implemented and monitored through contractual agreements with specialized providers of clinical services collectively known as contract research organizations (CROs)/site management organizations (SMOs) or Specialty Networks.

A. Contract Research Organizations and Site Management Organizations

What They Are and What They Do

In the past, pharmaceutical companies supervised their own clinical trials, from the discovery of the compound to animal testing to the preliminary testing of human subjects to the larger clinical trials involving hundreds or thousands of patients. To assist pharmaceutical companies, CROs/SMOs/Specialty Networks have developed to handle all of that and more.

CROs are composed of companies that run parts or all of the clinical trials. SMOs generally are a group of physicians and research professionals willing to offer their services to conduct the actual clinical trials. Specialty Networks are composed of sites in a specific medical specialty that not only perform clinical trials but also offer additional services assisting in the conduct of clinical trials. These organizations arose to fill a need: to assist the pharmaceutical companies in the drug development process. According to an article in the *New York Times* published in May 1999, these organizations evolved to elevate the enormous pressure that began around 1992 from managed care companies and health insurers on drug companies to hold down prices. The Food and Drug Administration (FDA) encouraged development of these companies in order to speed up its approval process. The average review time for new drug applications (NDAs) dropped from more than 22 months in 1990 to just over 14 months in 1997, according to the FDA.

Pharmaceutical companies found they had to invest more effort and revenue into finding drugs to develop, while at the same time cutting their development costs. For many pharmaceutical companies, the solution was to dismantle all or part of their clinical research monitoring departments that ran the clinical trials, turning the work over to smaller companies that had emerged to fill the industry's needs.

CROs can assist the pharmaceutical companies by:

- ✔ designing the Protocol, case report forms (CRFs), and source documents required for each clinical trial;

- ✔ locating Principal Investigators (PIs);

- ✔ assisting in potential patient recruitment efforts;

- ✔ statistically analyzing the clinical trial data;

- ✔ meeting with the FDA;

- ✔ preparing the enormous amount of paperwork required by the FDA for submission before the test article can be approved;

- ✔ writing the scientific papers for publication and presentation at national and international scientific meetings;

- ✔ conducting periodic auditing of Investigator sites to ensure the study is being conducted according to the Protocol, the Code of Federal Regulations, and Good Clinical Practice (GCP) guidelines;

- ✔ selecting and coordinating central laboratories; and

- ✔ selecting and coordinating Independent Institutional Review Boards (IRBs).

SMOs and Specialty Networks can assist the pharmaceutical industry by:

- ✔ providing a national network of physicians experienced in a specific therapeutic area (such as oncology, cardiology, and neurology) in conducting clinical trials;

- ✔ coordinating the completion of the required regulatory documents for their sites;

- ✔ providing technology to assist in the conduct of a clinical study;

- ✔ negotiating the budget for their sites;

- ✔ handling the financial aspects of the clinical trial for their sites, invoicing the Sponsor, and providing payment to their sites;

- ✔ providing ongoing training to their sites;

- ✔ providing tools for their sites to meet enrollment commitments;

- ✔ providing their sites with a set of standard operating procedures (SOPs);

- ✔ developing study-specific source documents for their sites; and

- ✔ providing data coordinators to assist in the completion of the CRFs.

In addition to providing these services, several organizations have a Phase I unit, on-site or off-site, where they can conduct clinical trials introducing the test article for the first time to healthy human subjects.

The size of these organizations varies from large corporations to groups of physicians conducting clinical trials in a specialized area such as oncology and urology to a rolodex of the names of physicians interested in participating in clinical trials to a directory of physicians by specialty to a website listing clinical trials seeking PIs to a company of one person working out of her/his home to assist in the clinical research process.

Due to the nature of clinical research, these organizations will continue to provide the pharmaceutical industry with the necessary support needed to conduct clinical trials. The CRC and PI play pivotal roles in ensuring the smooth conduct of a study. By understanding all elements of the clinical Protocol, the CRFs, and the study design, the CRC, PI, CROs/SMOs/Specialty Networks, and Sponsor will be able to work together to efficiently meet the study goals.

B. Good Clinical Practice Guidelines

What Is Good Clinical Practice?

GCP is a standard for the:

- ✔ Design
- ✔ Conduct
- ✔ Performance
- ✔ Monitoring
- ✔ Auditing
- ✔ Recording
- ✔ Analyses
- ✔ Reporting

of clinical trials.

GCP ensures the rights and safety of clinical trial subjects and the integrity of clinical data obtained during the conduct of a clinical trial. GCP concerns everyone working on *any* aspect of clinical research.

GCP guidelines were developed to ensure that only adequately planned and conducted clinical trials are performed in order to safeguard the interests of the patient, Investigator, Sponsor, and the general community.

What Is the International Conference on Harmonisation?

The International Conference on Harmonisation (ICH) is an international standard for the:

✔ Design

✔ Conduct

✔ Performance

✔ Monitoring

✔ Auditing

✔ Recording

✔ Analyses

✔ Reporting

that provides assurance that the clinical data obtained and reported results during the conduct of a clinical trial are credible and accurate and that the rights, integrity, and confidentiality of study subjects are protected.

Revised ICH Terms of Reference

✔ To maintain a forum for a constructive dialogue between regulatory authorities and the pharmaceutical industry on the real and perceived differences in the technical requirements for product registration in the European Union, United States, and Japan in order to ensure a more timely introduction of new medicinal product and their availability to patients

✔ To contribute to the protection of public health from an international perspective

✔ To monitor and update harmonized technical requirements leading to a greater mutual acceptance of research and development data

✔ To avoid divergent future requirements through harmonization of selected topics needed as a result of therapeutic advances and the development of new technologies for the production of medicinal products

✔ To facilitate the adoption of new or improved technical research and development approaches that update or replace current practices, where these permit a more economical use of human, animal, and material resources, without compromising safety

✔ To facilitate the dissemination and communication of information on harmonized guidelines and their use such as to encourage the implementation and integration of common standards

C. Declaration of Helsinki

The Declaration of Helsinki states:

- ✔ Research must conform to scientific principles.
- ✔ Protocols must be approved by an independent ethics committee.
- ✔ Clinical trials must be supervised and conducted by suitably qualified persons.
- ✔ Objectives and possible benefits must be balanced against the risk to the human subject.
- ✔ Privacy of the human subject must be respected, and there is minimal physical and mental impact on the subject.
- ✔ Informed consent must be obtained from a potential human subject prior to the performance of *any* study-related procedures.

D. Sponsor of a Clinical Trial

The Sponsor of a clinical trial is an individual or organization responsible for the initiation, management, and/or financing of clinical trials. The Sponsor of a clinical trial is generally the organization that possesses permission from the appropriate regulatory agency to conduct the clinical trial. In most instances, the Sponsor is a pharmaceutical company.

Sponsor responsibilities include:

- ✔ Providing the investigational study trial material
- ✔ Providing technology to assist in the conduct of a clinical study
- ✔ Providing a Protocol and ensuring Protocol compliance
- ✔ Providing monitoring and source data verification
- ✔ Maintaining study trial material disposition records
- ✔ Data management
- ✔ Record retention of the study-related documents
- ✔ Providing compensation and indemnity for clinical trial-related injury
- ✔ Assuring the quality of the clinical trial data

IV. Investigator Responsibilities

A. Condensed Version

Administrative

- ✔ Review Protocol, Investigator Brochure, conventions, associated documents

- ✔ Communication with Institutional Review Board (IRB)

- ✔ Hospital management (in-patient study)

- ✔ Curriculum vitae/medical or professional license

- ✔ Informed consent

- ✔ Records and reports

- ✔ Delegation of tasks specific to the clinical trial

Logistics

- ✔ Sufficient time to conduct study/adequate staff/appropriate facilities

- ✔ Ensure all research staff adequately informed on all aspects of the Protocol

- ✔ List of delegated study-related tasks and the names of those qualified to perform the tasks

Study Drug Management

- ✔ Full study drug accountability documentation

  - Receipt of the investigational product

- ✔ Inventory, return, disposition of the investigational product

  - Properly used by patients

- ✔ Safe and proper handling and secure storage of the investigational product

- ✔ Ensure patient compliance with the investigational product

- ✔ Randomization procedures conducted according to the Protocol
- ✔ Unblinding procedures conducted according to the Protocol
  - • Disclosure envelopes containing study drug/placebo information
  - • Emergency situation

Informed Consent

- ✔ Informed consent must be approved by an IRB
- ✔ Must be obtained prior to the performance of any study-related procedure and documented in the clinical records
- ✔ Consent obtained in writing
- ✔ Use of correct version of the informed consent
- ✔ Signed and personally dated by the patient or the patient's legal representative
- ✔ Provide copy of the fully executed informed consent to the patient
- ✔ Inform the patient if there is any new information that may impact the patient's continued participation in the study

INFORMED CONSENT IS A PROCESS—NOT JUST A WRITTEN DOCUMENT.

Safety Reporting

- ✔ Adverse events/laboratory abnormalities
- ✔ Expedited reporting

Data Collection

- ✔ Case report forms (CRFs) completed properly, entirely, and in a timely manner
- ✔ Make data available for monitoring audit
- ✔ Indicate ongoing review of subjects labs and procedure reports by dating and initialing when reviewed

B. Clinical Trial Monitoring of Documentation

Purpose of monitoring:

- ✔ To verify that informed consent was obtained prior to the conduct of any study-related procedures
- ✔ To verify the study is conducted strictly according to the Protocol
- ✔ To verify the study subjects have met the inclusion and exclusion criteria and, if applicable, to verify an enrollment waiver was granted by the appropriate

study personnel and a copy of the waiver signed by the person granting the waiver is on file at the site

✔ To verify all primary and secondary efficacy variables

✔ To review all pertinent patient safety information, including serious adverse events (SAEs), adverse events (AEs), and study procedures being followed according to the Protocol, and to document if any Protocol procedures are not being followed (e.g., study procedures not being performed) and if any patients were enrolled into the clinical trial without meeting the inclusion/exclusion criteria and did not obtain a waiver from the appropriate study personnel

✔ To verify the study drug is being stored, dispensed, and returned correctly and that appropriate study drug accountability records are being maintained

✔ To verify that the information contained in the CRFs is accurate and verifiable with source documentation

C. Investigator Responsibilities

When a Principal Investigator (PI) signs the form FDA 1572, he/she makes the following legal commitments to the Food and Drug Administration (FDA):

1. Agrees to conduct the study(ies) in accordance with the relevant, current Protocol(s) and will only make changes in a Protocol *after* notifying the Sponsor, except when necessary to protect the safety, rights, or welfare of subjects.

2. Agrees to *personally* conduct or supervise the described investigation(s).

3. Agrees to inform any patient or any person used as controls that the drugs are being used for investigational purposes and will ensure that the requirements relating to obtaining informed consent in 21 CFR Part 50 and IRB review and approval in 21 CFR Part 56 are met.

4. Agrees to report to the Sponsor adverse experiences that occur in the course of the investigation(s) in accordance with 21 CFR Part 312.64.

5. Acknowledges understanding of the information in the Investigator Brochure, including the potential risks and side effects of the drug.

6. Agrees to ensure that all associates, colleagues, and employees assisting in the conduct of the study(ies) are informed about their obligations in meeting these stated commitments.

7. Agrees to maintain adequate and accurate records in accordance with 21 CFR 312.62 and to make those records available for inspection in accordance with 21 CFR 312.68.

8. Ensures that an IRB that complies with the requirements of 21 CRF Part 56 will be responsible for the initial and continuing review and approval of the clinical investigation.

9. Agrees to promptly report to the IRB all changes in the research activity and all unanticipated problems involving risks to human subjects.

10. Agrees to not make any changes in the research Protocol without IRB approval, except when necessary to eliminate apparent immediate hazards to human subjects.

11. Agrees to comply with all other requirements regarding the obligations of clinical investigators and all other pertinent requirements in 21 CFR Part 312.

These commitments are considered essential to the success of a clinical trial in accordance with FDA regulations and Good Clinical Practice (GCP) and International Conference on Harmonisation (ICH) guidelines.

Useful reference: FDA Compliance Program Guidance Manual (7348.811) "Clinical Investigators"

Principal Investigator

The PI of a clinical trial must be qualified by education and training in the therapeutic area of the clinical trial being conducted by the applicable regulatory requirements (Code of Federal Regulations, GCP and ICH Guidelines). The PI must maintain a current medical license (e.g., MD, DO, DPM) and sometimes advanced training (Board Certified) for trials in specialty therapeutic areas. The PI must be familiar with the investigational product being used in the clinical trial and must also comply with the applicable regulatory requirements.

The PI is ultimately responsible for the conduct of a clinical study at a trial site as well as the integrity, health, and welfare of the human subjects during the clinical trial.

Principal Investigator Responsibilities

The responsibilities of the PI include:

- ✔ Obtaining informed consent from a patient prior to the performance of *any* study-related procedures, including documentation in the patient's clinical chart that written informed consent was obtained prior to the performance of any study-related procedures

- ✔ Ensuring the informed consent document was approved by an IRB and the correct version of the informed consent is being used

- ✔ Complying with the IRB-approved Protocol

- ✔ Maintaining study trial material accountability

✔ Medically supervising the conduct of the clinical trial

✔ Maintaining adequate patient records and CRFs

✔ Maintaining the site facilities and staff and ensuring both are adequate to perform the study-related procedures

✔ Enrolling the adequate number of study patients required by the Sponsor

✔ Ensuring adequate reporting of AEs and SAEs to the IRBs or Ethics Committees according to Federal Regulations

✔ Archiving study-related documents for the time period required by the Sponsor or Regulatory Authorities

Principal Investigator Responsibilities and Informed Consent

The PI, or a qualified person designated by the PI, should fully inform the potential subject of all pertinent aspects of the clinical trial. Documentation of these discussions is necessary to ensure study-related procedures were not performed prior to the signing of the informed consent document. The informed consent document must be signed, dated, and witnessed by an unbiased third party. GCP and ICH guidelines sometimes allow a subject to be entered into a trial without a signed informed consent form but only in special limited circumstances. Some institutions also require the approval of an independent "Ombudsman" to review and approve a subject's enrollment in certain risky trials. Finally, in trials involving children, permission must be obtained from the parents or guardians, and adequate provisions must be made for obtaining the assent of children if they are younger than 18 but above the age of reason (usually about 7 years old).

Who Should Administer Informed Consent?

ICH 4.8.5 states "The Investigator, or a person designated by the Investigator, should fully inform the subject ..."

ICH 2.1 states "Clinical trials should be conducted in accordance with the ethical principles that have their origin in the Declaration of Helsinki ..."

Declaration of Helsinki B (21) states, "The physician should then obtain the subject's freely-given informed consent ..."

The ultimate responsibility of administering informed consent still resides with the PI. An auditor would expect the required documentation, reassurance that the PI is knowledgeable, and that a physician or qualified medical professional was available at the time of consent, if applicable, to answer a subject's medically related questions. In addition, in the documentation in the potential clinical trial subject's chart, there must be proof that consent was obtained prior to performing any study-related procedures. The entry should note the time the informed consent was obtained, providing reassurance that informed consent was obtained correctly.

Adhering to the Approved Study Protocol

A PI conducting clinical trials must adhere to the approved study Protocol. The PI ensures that the Protocol and amendments are strictly followed. The PI agrees not to make any changes to the study procedures without prior agreement of the Sponsor and the IRB, except when necessary to eliminate apparent immediate hazard to a study subject. The PI documents and explains any deviation from the approved Protocol and the reason for the deviation. If a study procedure is not conducted according to the Protocol, it is generally considered a Protocol violation. If, prior to the study procedure deviation, permission is given from the Sponsor and/or Study Medical Monitor, it is frequently considered a waiver. For instance, Patient #0003 did not return to the clinic for Protocol-specific procedures and did not notify the PI. If this omission was noted during a regular monitoring visit, it would be considered to be a Protocol violation. However, if this same patient were to inform the PI he/she would not be able to return to the clinic on the specified day for Protocol-specific procedures and the PI contacted the Sponsor and/or the Medical Monitor, a waiver could be granted. There can be no waiver or Protocol exception for a deviation from the Protocol *after* it has occurred. This is one reason communication between the PI, the PI's staff, the Monitor, and the Sponsor is of critical importance.

Study Drug Accountability

The PI is ultimately responsible for maintaining study drug accountability. All study medications must be stored in a secured location accessible by the PI, or assigned pharmacist, or assigned study staff such as the CRC, and it is a good practice to isolate study drugs from marketed drugs. The PI and/or a pharmacist or other designated study personnel must maintain current records of the product's delivery to the site. This record includes the product's inventory at the site, the use by each subject, and the return of the used/returned or unused products to the Sponsor or alternate disposition of the unused product(s). ***It is important to note: Returned/dispensed study products should not be stored as study drug has not yet been dispensed to a subject.***

Study Drug Accountability Records are maintained to include the dates, quantities, batch/serial numbers, expiry dates, and unique code numbers. It is important to provide instructions for the correct use of the study drug. It is also important to remember that the Study Coordinator or the pharmacist may dispense study medication only under the supervision of the PI or subinvestigator listed on the FDA 1572.

If the study drug is transported from one satellite center to another location, (if applicable) it is important to have a written policy and a procedure in place to document that the integrity of the study drug was maintained during the transporting. *Prior* approval must be obtained from the Sponsor before the study drug is transported from one center to another. Some centers have forms in place that document the date, time, and person transporting the study drug as well as document the date, time, and name of the person receiving the study drug. If the study drug requires refrigeration (36–46° F) or controlled room temperature (59–86° F), then appropriate storage measures must be taken to ensure the required temperature is maintained during transport and must be documented to protect the integrity of the study drug.

The study drug should only be dispensed to the person actually taking the medication. It is not acceptable for a spouse, friend, or relative to pick up the study drug for a patient. It is also usually a study requirement that the study patient returns the unused study medication (including the package) before additional study drug is dispensed. In rare instances, this may not be possible; however, it would be a good idea to contact the Monitor or Sponsor prior to dispensing the medication in order to obtain a waiver if applicable.

Medical Supervision of the Clinical Trial

The PI must be responsible for all study-related medical decisions; this includes the supervision of all AEs, dose changes, and discussions with the study patient about intercurrent illnesses.

The PI must maintain adequate patient records, which should include the following:

✔ Patient demographics.

✔ Date of the study visit or unscheduled visit.

✔ Documentation that the patient consented to participate in the clinical trial and that no study-related procedures were performed prior to obtaining the informed consent. It is also a good practice to note in the chart or medical record the time consent was obtained.

✔ Patient eligibility and verification. The PI or subinvestigator should confirm in writing that the patient has met the inclusion/exclusion criteria required by the Protocol prior to receiving study medication.

✔ Concomitant medications and the indications for the medication. It is a good practice to make sure the medication the patient is taking does not conflict with the patient's medical history prior to dispensing the study medication.

✔ Documentation of all AEs reported by the patient as required by the Protocol, especially SAEs, i.e., those requiring hospitalization.

✔ Appropriate HIPAA documentation. All patient information is confidential.

Maintaining Adequate Site Facilities and Staff

The PI should have available an adequate number of qualified staff members and adequate facilities for the foreseeable duration of the clinical trial. This would include calibration of equipment used during the study and the retention of equipment service records. The PI also ensures all staff members assisting with the clinical trial are adequately trained and knowledgeable about the

Protocol, the procedures, and the investigational product(s), and the staff person's role and responsibilities in the clinical trial.

Maintaining Adequate Number of Study Subjects

The PI should be able to demonstrate a potential for recruiting the required number of qualified study subjects eligible to participate in the clinical trial within the agreed recruitment period. In addition, the PI must have sufficient time to properly conduct and complete the clinical trial within the agreed clinical trial period. No extended vacations or sabbaticals should occur before the end of the trial.

Investigator Responsibilities

The PI is responsible for reporting AEs and SAEs experienced by subjects participating in a clinical trial. The PI must immediately inform the Sponsor of any serious or unexpected AE occurring during the clinical trial. The PI must notify the IRB or Independent Ethics Committee of these events. All serious AEs are accompanied by an assessment of causality and possible impact on the clinical trial. It is not appropriate to delegate this responsibility to the Study Coordinator or the research nurse, regardless of their experience. This is a function that must be performed by the PI or the subinvestigator.

Archiving Study Documents

The PI must retain records and data from the clinical trial for safety reasons and for audit and inspection subsequent to study completion. The records must be maintained in a secure area in order to prevent undue access, loss, or tampering. Unless specified in the Protocol, the study records must be maintained for no less than 15 years. In some cases the issue of product liability may dictate longer retention time by Sponsors. The Sponsors usually send written notification when the study files may be discarded.

As a Principal Investigator, it is important to remember that you can delegate a task—but never the responsibility.

V. Duties of the Clinical Research Coordinator

The CRC or research nurse plays a pivotal role in the efficient progress of the clinical study. The CRC is often responsible for organizing the documentation and files pertaining to a study and for coordinating the subsequent activities of the investigators and subjects. The responsibilities of the CRC will vary at each investigational site, but may include the following:

✔ To review and familiarize themselves and other staff with the Protocol

✔ To provide prospective investigators with a copy of the Protocol

✔ To notify the Sponsor and CRO/SMO/Specialty Network of investigators' interest in participating in the study

✔ To prepare a grant (if needed) in conjunction with the Sponsor

✔ To compile the required information for the Sponsor and CRO/SMO/Specialty Network

✔ To review FDA requirements and ICH and GCP guidelines

✔ To prepare for the IRB meeting, including preparation of the informed consent document (to be forwarded to the Sponsor before the IRB meeting) and other prestudy documentation, preparation of the meeting agenda, and mailing of the IRB meeting notice to investigators

✔ To attend the IRB meeting and to have proposed IRB approval letters ready (both the PI and the CRC should attend, if possible)

✔ To identify the study site's contact person

✔ To establish the need for a Letter of Indemnification from the Sponsor

✔ To schedule on-site visits with the Sponsor

✔ To participate in the Investigator meeting

✔ To prepare additional study records, forms, and letters as directed by the CRO/SMO/Specialty Network or Sponsor

✔ To set up study files

✔ To enroll subjects

✔ To oversee study activities, including the secure storage of the test article

✔ To maintain accurate and complete records

✔ To close the study with the Sponsor and to store the study records appropriately

A. Compiling Prestudy Documents

Before subjects can be enrolled in a study and before test articles can be shipped, several prestudy documents must be compiled by the CRC or Investigator and sent for approval to the Sponsor. Descriptions of these documents follow.

Form FDA 1572. This is the Statement of Investigator form, which summarizes what the FDA requires for an acceptable clinical study. It must be signed by the PI. In addition, all subinvestigators (if any) who are participating in the study and who are authorized to administer the test articles must be listed. In most instances, the Sponsor determines which study personnel are required on the Form FDA 1572. The actual form, along with a sample of a completed version, is provided in Appendix II (Form 2). Investigators who sign Form FDA 1572 make the following commitments:

✔ To conduct the study according to the Protocol (Changes made to the Protocol can be made after notification to the sponsoring pharmaceutical company, except to protect patient safety. Investigators who deviate from the Protocol for any reason need also to notify their IRB in writing of the deviation.)

✔ To personally conduct and/or supervise the research Protocol

✔ To inform patients that they are participating in a research study

✔ To abide by the IRB and informed consent regulations

✔ To report all SAEs according to Federal Regulations to the sponsoring pharmaceutical company and the IRB

✔ To read and understand the Investigator Brochure for the investigational material being tested

✔ To ensure that other personnel involved with the study meet these commitments

✔ To maintain accurate study records and to make these records available for inspection by the appropriate agencies (FDA and the sponsoring pharmaceutical company and their representatives)

✔ To ensure initial and continuing review and approval of the research study by the IRB

✔ To comply with the Federal Regulations for investigators in 21 CFR 312

Note: The PI may delegate some of these responsibilities to the CRC, but, ultimately, the PI is responsible for ensuring that they are done correctly.

Curricula Vitae (CV). These are required of the PI and all the subinvestigators listed on Form FDA 1572. Curricula vitae should be updated every two years, and they should be signed and dated to show that they are current. A copy of the physician's medical license as well as proof of malpractice insurance may be required by some sponsors. In addition, CVs of the CRC and the laboratory director, if appropriate (i.e., when a central laboratory is used by a Sponsor), may also be required.

Lab Certification. A copy of the laboratory license, laboratory certification, and the normal laboratory values for the laboratory to be used must be on file.

Signed Protocol. This must be signed and dated by the PI, along with any Protocol amendments.

Financial Certification/Disclosure. The following are the necessary financial certification/disclosure requirements:

✔ Every PI needs to certify/disclose if he/she has a financial interest in the sponsoring pharmaceutical company or in the investigational material being tested.

✔ Certification is required for each PI and all subinvestigators listed on Form FDA 1572.

✔ This certification encompasses not only the Investigator, but also his/her spouse and each dependent child.

✔ The certification is applicable for the time during which the PI is conducting the study and for one year following completion of the study (i.e., after enrollment of all subjects and follow-up subjects, in accordance with the Protocol). The sponsoring pharmaceutical company should be notified in writing of any change in the accuracy of the certification during the clinical trial.

✔ Any financial interest in the sponsoring pharmaceutical company or in the product being tested needs to be promptly disclosed to the sponsoring pharmaceutical company.

Specifically, each PI must certify/disclose that he/she:

✔ has not entered into any financial arrangement with the sponsoring pharmaceutical company, whereby the outcome of the clinical study could affect his/her compensation (e.g., bonus, royalty, or other financial incentive);

✔ does not have a proprietary interest in the study material (e.g., patent, trademark, copyright, licensing agreement, etc.);

✔ does not have a significant equity interest in the sponsoring pharmaceutical company, not applicable to the material being tested; and

✔ has not received significant payments or money or anything of value from the sponsoring pharmaceutical company with a value in excess of $25,000, other than payments for conducting the clinical study (e.g., grants, compensation in the form of equipment, retainers for ongoing consultation and honoraria paid to the investigator or to the institution in support of the PI's activities).

Other documents that are required to be on file before a study may begin include the IRB approval and membership list, the budget for the study, the Letter of Agreement between the Sponsor and CRO/SMO or Investigator, and the approved informed consent form. The Sponsor will inform the CRC of the documents needed at each step of the study. The Administrative Checklist (see Appendix II, Form 6) provides a mechanism to determine if appropriate documentation has been obtained and completed.

B. Creating and Maintaining Study Files

The Study File. Once all prestudy documents have been compiled, the Study File should be created. This file will be maintained throughout the clinical study and will eventually contain samples of all forms and reports to be completed during the course of the study, in addition to all prestudy documents.

Initially, the following materials should be included in the Study File:

✔ Prestudy documents, including:

  ✔ Form FDA 1572;

  ✔ current, signed, and dated (within two years) CV of investigators, CRC, and laboratory director;

  ✔ current medical license;

  ✔ proof of malpractice insurance (if required);

  ✔ Financial disclosure form;

  ✔ Investigational New Drug (IND) Application, safety letters, if applicable;

- ✔ Protocol specific training;

- ✔ current laboratory certification and normal ranges for laboratory values;

- ✔ Protocol (including signature page and synopsis), including amendments to the Protocol;

- ✔ current IRB membership list;

- ✔ IRB approval;

- ✔ IRB-approved informed consent form;

- ✔ IRB-approved advertising, including any written information provided to a subject during the study;

- ✔ Investigator Brochure (all versions);

- ✔ Test Article Inventory and Drug Accountability Record;

- ✔ Completed and signed Delegation of Responsibilities form;

- ✔ CRFs and Adverse Experience forms;

- ✔ Completed and signed Authorized Representative Signature Record;

- ✔ Specimen Submission Records (if required);

- ✔ Site visit log;

- ✔ Telephone log;

- ✔ IRB fee letter;

- ✔ Letter of Indemnification; and

- ✔ all correspondence to and from Sponsor.

Financial records, with the exception of the completed financial disclosure forms, should not be filed in the Study File. Protocol specific financial records should be filed separately from the Study File. The clinical research associate (CRA) will review the Study File with the CRC at the beginning of the study to ensure that all of the required documentation is present.

As the study progresses, additional documents will be completed. These (or copies) should be retained in the Study File. Examples include:

- ✔ amendments to the Protocol;

- ✔ executed informed consent forms;

- ✔ laboratory test results;

- ✔ shipping invoices for all test articles, Returned Goods form/destruction forms, if applicable;

- ✔ ongoing correspondence;
- ✔ other source documents;
- ✔ miscellaneous Sponsor forms;
- ✔ revised informed consent forms; and
- ✔ correspondence to and from the IRB regarding the progress of the study, Protocol deviations, and submission of IND Safety Reports.

If a copy of a form is kept in another file, the original should be readily available and its location should be noted in a memo to the Investigator File.

The Subject Workfolder. Subject Workfolders must also be compiled for each subject enrolled in the study. When correctly organized, these greatly facilitate the proper collection of study data and form the core of the clinical database. Each Workfolder should contain the following, as appropriate:

- ✔ study design flow chart;
- ✔ screening sheet (inclusion/exclusion criteria);
- ✔ informed consent form (two signed copies—one for the research chart and one for the subject);
- ✔ laboratory requisitions packet;
- ✔ data collection form from CRF;
- ✔ specimen labels;
- ✔ Protocol specific procedures, i.e., ECG, chest x-ray;
- ✔ disbursement requests (compensation vouchers);
- ✔ a "STOP!—Research Subject" sign (see Appendix II, Forms 16 and 17);
- ✔ clinic notes;
- ✔ synopsis of Protocol;
- ✔ letters to the subject;
- ✔ demographic information, including a copy of the subject's photo identification if required;
- ✔ worksheet for outside departments; and
- ✔ Medical Release of Information for medical records.

Each document in the Subject Workfolder should be identified with a unique subject number. For example, 103A-207 may indicate Protocol 103A, site number 2, patient number 7.

The Audit File. At the conclusion of a study, an Audit File will be created. This will contain portions of the Study File, including:

✔ Site visit log;

✔ Telephone log;

✔ Protocol (all versions, including amendments);

✔ Informed consent form (all versions used during the study);

✔ Drug receipt/return log/destruction form, if applicable;

✔ Subject drug dispensation log;

✔ prestudy documents;

✔ correspondence; and

✔ Financial disclosure form (See Appendix II, Form 14).

C. Obtaining CLIA Laboratory Certification as It Pertains to Clinical Research

CLIA. The Clinical Lab Improvement Amendments (CLIA) of 1988 is a federal program established by Congress to improve the quality and reliability of clinical labs. CLIA requires that all clinical labs be certified through the Health Care Financing Administration (HCFA). HCFA is a division of the U.S. Department of Health and Human Services (DHHS). The DHHS in each state administers the CLIA program for their own state; however, lab certificates are issued through HCFA and are signed by an authorized HCFA representative. You will see a CLIA certificate sample later in the module.

Types of CLIA Certificates

The following are different types of CLIA certificates and can be issued to a lab upon inspection, depending on the types of testing it performs:

✔ Laboratory Certificate of Registration

✔ Laboratory Certificate of Compliance

✔ Laboratory Certificate of Accreditation

✔ Laboratory Certificate of Provider-Performed Microscopy Procedures (PPMP)

✔ Laboratory Certificate of Waiver

The following chart lists the three types of test classifications (types of test performed by a lab) and acceptable certificates for each classification. You must be familiar with the types of tests and acceptable certificates in order to verify that each lab has appropriate CLIA documentation while conducting a clinical trial.

Acceptable CLIA Certificates	
Test Classification	**Certificate(s) Required**

Moderate-to-Highly Complex Tests	CLIA Laboratory Certificate of Compliance
	
	OR
	
	Private Agency Certificate of Accreditation and a CLIA Laboratory Certficate of Accreditation
	
	• Whether a test is moderate or highly complex is dependent on the number of manual steps involved in completing the test and the level of interpretation required. For example, highly complex tests involve several critical steps and a high level of interpretation.
	
	Examples of moderately complex tests include:
	  – Liver enzymes
	  – Electrolytes
	  – PT / PTT
	
	Examples of highly complex tests include:
	  – HIV testing
	  – Manual cell counts
	  – DNA PCR tests
	  – Electrophoresis

Microscopy Procedures	CLIA Laboratory Certificate of Provider-Performed Microscopy Procedures • Microscopies include substances that a physician views under the microscope. For example, vaginal smears and semen.
Waived Tests	CLIA Laboratory Certificate of Waiver • Waived tests are laboratory examinations and procedures that have been approved by the FDA for home use or have been determined to be simple laboratory examinations and procedures that have an insignificant risk of an erroneous result.

Example of waived tests include:

- Dipstick or tablet reagent urinalysis (nonautomated) for bilirubin, glucose, ketones, hemoglobin, specific gravity, leukocytes, nitrates, protein, pH, and urobilinogen
- Fecal occult blood
- Ovulation test—visual color comparison test for human luteinizing hormone
- Urine prenancy test—visual color comparison tests
- Erythrocyte sedimentation rate (nonautomated)
- Blood glucose by blood glucose monitoring devices cleared by the FDA specifically for home use
- Spun microhematocrit

CLIA Certificate Descriptions

Now that you are familiar with the types of CLIA certificates, let us take a closer look at each one.

CLIA Certificate	Description
Laboratory Certificate of Registration	• Every lab that applies for a Certificate of Compliance or a Certificate of Accreditation receives this certificate. • Each lab is assigned a CLIA ID#—this number appears on all CLIA certificates. • This certificate indicates that the lab is registered with the HCFA through the State Department of Health—it **does not** indicate that the lab is in compliance with Federal CLIA requirements. • Laboratories applying for a Certificate of Compliance or a Certificate of Accreditation operate under the Certificate of Registration until the State Department of Health completes an inspection of the lab.

	• If the inspection is not conducted within 1 year, HCFA will renew the certificate for 1 more year, until the inspection is performed.
Laboratory Certificate of Compliance	• This certificate is issued to labs conducting moderate-to-highly complex testing. • The certificate is issued by HCFA after the State Department of Health has inspected the lab. • Labs operate under the Certificate of Registration until they receive the Certificate of Compliance. • Labs with this certificate can also perform microscopy procedures and waived tests. • The Certificate of Compliance is a stand-alone document.
Laboratory Certificate of Accreditation	• This certificate is issued to labs conducting moderate-to-highly complex testing. • After the lab contacts an approved Private Accrediting Agency, the agency conducts an inspection. If the lab passes inspection, the Private Accrediting Agency will issue its Certificate of Accreditation. • The Private Accrediting Agency notifies HCFA that the lab passed inspection. • HCFA then issues a CLIA Laboratory Certificate of Accreditation based on inspection results. • Labs operate under the Certificate of Registration until they receive the Certificate of Accreditation. • Labs with this certificate can also perform microscopy procedures and waived tests. • The Certificate of Accreditation **is not** a stand-alone document. The CLIA Certificate of Accreditation must be accompanied by the Certificate of Accreditation issued by the Private Accrediting Agency.
Laboratory Certificate of Provider-Performed Microscopy Procedures	• This certificate is issued to labs that perform microscopy procedures.

	• The certificate **does not** require an inspection. However, labs can be subject to an inspection if a complaint about them is made to the State Department of Health. • Labs applying for a Certificate of Provider-Performed Microscopy Procedures **do not** receive a CLIA Certificate of Registration. • A lab with this certificate can also perform waived tests. • The Certificate of Provider-Performed Microscopy Procedures is a stand-alone document.
Laboratory Certificate of Waiver	• This certificate is issued to labs that only perform waived tests. • Labs that only perform waived tests are waived from routine inspections, proficiency testing, quality assurance, quality control, and lab personnel requirements. • The certificate does not require an inspection. However, labs can be subject to an inspection if a complaint about them is made to the State Department of Health. • Labs applying for a Certificate of Waiver **do not** receive a CLIA Certificate of Registration. • The Certificate of Waiver is a stand-alone document.

It can take several months for HCFA to issue a CLIA Laboratory Certificate. If the certificate expires during the conduct of a clinical trial and the lab director has applied for a Certificate of Registration but has not yet received it:

> ✔ Ask the lab for its CLIA ID#.

> ✔ Ask the lab to provide you with a letter of notification from its State Department of Health. This letter should acknowledge that the lab has applied for CLIA certification and should include their CLIA ID#.

CLIA Certificate Sample

The following page shows a sample of a CLIA Laboratory Certificate of Accreditation. Note that the certificate has some important key elements. The certificate:

```
Department of Health & Human Services

Health Care Financing Administration

Laboratory:              Clinical Labs, Inc.        CLIA ID#:  07D0092519

Mailing Address:         4321 Stanton St.
                         Cincinnati, OH 55155       Effective Date:    October 2004

Laboratory Director:     John Ninane               Expiration Date:   November 2006

Physical Location:       4321 Stanton St.
                         Cincinnati, OH 55155

              CLIA LABORATORY CERTIFICATE OF ACCREDITATION

Pursuant to Section 353 of the Public Health Service Act (42 U.S.C.263a) as revised by the Clinical Laboratory Improvement Amendments (CLIA), Public
Law 110-578, the above named laboratory located at the address shown hereon (and other locations registered under this certificate) is hereby authorized to
accept human specimens for the purposes of performing laboratory examinations.

This certificate shall be valid until the expiration date above, but is subject revocation, suspension, limitation, or other sanctions for violations of the Act or
the regulations promulgated thereunder.



                                           John J. Sullivan, Director
                                           Division of Laboratories and Acute Care Services
                                           Survey and Certification Group
                                           Center for Medicaid and State Operations
```

✔ Is issued under the name "Department of Health & Human Services—Health Care Financing Administration"

✔ Lists the name and address of the lab

✔ Lists the name of the lab director

✔ Contains the lab's CLIA ID#

✔ Clearly identifies the type of certificate

✔ Indicates the expiration date for the certificate

✔ Is signed by an authorized HCFA representative

Private Accreditation Agencies

As mentioned earlier, laboratories performing moderate-to-highly complex tests must be certified through the HCFA. Laboratories have the choice to apply for either a CLIA Laboratory Certificate of Compliance or a CLIA Laboratory Certificate of Accreditation. If the lab chooses to apply for a CLIA Laboratory Certificate of Accreditation, the laboratory will not be inspected by the State Department of Health but by a Private Accreditation Agency. The Private Accreditation Agency must be approved by the HCFA, which means that the HCFA has deemed the accreditation program to meet CLIA statutory requirements.

The following is a list of private agencies that have been approved by HCFA:

- ✔ Joint Commission on Accreditation of Healthcare Organizations (JCAHO)
- ✔ American Osteopathic Association (AOA)
- ✔ American Association of Blood Banks (AABB)
- ✔ College of American Pathologists (CAP)
- ✔ Commission on Office Laboratory Accreditation (COLA)
- ✔ American Society of Histocompatibility and Immunogenetics (ASHI)

Other than CLIA certificates, CAP certificates are the ones most commonly provided. It can take up to six months for CAP to issue an accreditation certificate. When CAP certifies a lab, it notifies HCFA. HCFA then issues a CLIA Laboratory Certificate of Accreditation.

CLIA Exemptions

HCFA recognizes some states as having equal or more stringent laws than CLIA. Labs that are licensed in the following states are exempt from CLIA requirements:

- ✔ New York is partially exempt. While commercial laboratories and hospital laboratories are not required to be CLIA certified, private physician office laboratories are required. Therefore, New York is partially exempt from CLIA. For example, if an Investigator in New York is performing a urine pregnancy test required per Protocol, the Investigator must have a CLIA Laboratory Certificate of Waiver.
- ✔ Washington

Veterans Affairs (VA) Medical Centers are also exempt from CLIA.

CLIA waives certification requirements for the following situations because they do not treat subjects based on the lab results

- ✔ Any laboratory that conducts testing solely for forensic purposes
- ✔ Research laboratories that test human specimens, but do not report any patient-specific results for the diagnosis, treatment, or assessment of the health of individual patients
- ✔ Individuals (for example, home health agency employees) who assist patients in their home with testing kits approved by the FDA
- ✔ Entities that serve as collection stations for specimens but send specimens to a certified lab for analysis

Documentation of the proper laboratory license and certifications are critical to the conduct of a clinical trial at a site.

VI. The Creation of Study Source Documents

Documentation of clinical research projects is undeniably one of the most important aspects of conducting a clinical study; yet, it is one of the major deficiencies repeatedly found by FDA auditors. A common source of disagreements about what constitutes source documentation continues to be an ongoing dialogue between Sponsors'/CROs'/SMOs' monitors and site personnel. Source documents confirm that the data were accurately reported and that the study was conducted according to the Protocol.

The Code of Federal Regulations and ICH and GCP guidelines require the following:

1. written, informed consent by all subjects **prior** to the implementation of any study-related procedures; and

2. accurate, complete, and appropriate clinical research documentation.

A. Source Documents—What Are They?

The first recording of any observations made or data generated about a study subject during his/her participation in a clinical trial is source documentation. Source documentation is the foundation of all clinical studies. Source documents confirm the completeness and accuracy of data collection and show evidence that the study was conducted not only according to the Protocol but also ethically.

CFR 312.62 (b) states "An investigator is required to prepare and maintain adequate and accurate case histories that record all observations and other data pertinent to the investigation on each individual administered the investigational drug or employed as a control in the investigation. Case histories include the CRFs and supporting data including, for example, signed and dated consent forms and medical records, including, for example, progress notes of the physician, the individual's hospital chart(s), and the nurses' notes."

ICH GCP 1.52 states "Source documents are the original documents, data, and records (e.g., hospital records; clinical and office charts; laboratory notes; memoranda; subjects' diaries or evaluation checklist; pharmacy dispensing records; recorded data from automated instruments; copies or transcriptions certified and verification of their accuracy; microfiches; photographic negatives; microfilm or magnetic media; x-rays; subject files; and records kept at the pharmacy, at the laboratories, and at medico-technical departments involved in the clinical trial)."

Copies of the CRFs *are not* source documents unless specifically identified by the Sponsor. *The sponsoring pharmaceutical companies' CROs/SMOs have been providing clinical research sites with source documents that are study-specific.* While this helps the CRC, generally it is better to create source documents that are study-specific and to mirror the information in the CRFs and reflect the standard operating procedures (SOPs) at the site.

Anyone involved in the clinical study can create source documents. This may include, but is not limited to, the PI, subinvestigators, CRC, floor nurse (if an in-patient study), physical therapist, data coordinator, and so forth. The pharmacist who records the dispensing of the study drug creates a source document. A research subject can create source documents when he/she completes study-specific diaries.

B. Source Document Examples

- ✔ a record release form with the subject's signature and date;
- ✔ completed and signed HIPAA consent, if applicable;
- ✔ letter of referral from the subject's primary physician to the PI for study screening;
- ✔ screening or intake forms;
- ✔ medical history, including demographic data and documentation of inclusion/exclusion eligibility;
- ✔ original, signed, and dated informed consent form;
- ✔ amendments to the original informed consent form, signed and dated;
- ✔ physical exam notes;
- ✔ progress notes;
- ✔ study-specific flow sheets;
- ✔ study-specific checklists;
- ✔ AE list;
- ✔ subject diaries;
- ✔ nurse's notes;
- ✔ Medication Administration Records (MARs);
- ✔ concomitant medication list;
- ✔ hospital admission and discharge summaries;
- ✔ certified copies of electronic medical records;
- ✔ correspondence to and from a study subject; and
- ✔ death certificate.

C. Types of Medical Reports
Generated While a Subject Is Enrolled in a Study

- ✔ laboratory: serology, chemistry, hematology, microbiology, urinalysis;
- ✔ ECG reports;
- ✔ MRI/CT scan reports;

✔ radiology reports;

✔ pathology reports;

✔ transfusion records;

✔ hospital admission summaries; and

✔ hospital discharge summaries.

Source documents should be accurate and complete enough to permit the entire reconstruction of the data in the unlikely event of losing the CRF. Information pertinent to the subject's participation in the study should be included. Variables, such as safety data and essential effectiveness, will determine the outcome of the clinical trial and should be documented. AEs, treatment, and follow-up should be described well. All communication with the Sponsor/CRO/SMO regarding approved Protocol waivers or deviations should be noted. (The IRB should be notified in writing of any waivers or deviations from the approved Protocol.)

It has been reported by experienced CRCs that every hour spent with a study subject generally requires at least an additional hour spent documenting and completing paperwork associated with the interaction. Documentation should be practical, limited to the essential, easy to routinize, and standardized but flexible enough to include unusual circumstances.

D. Good Clinical Research Documentation Details

✔ There should be a record of every visit and conversation with the subject in the subject's clinic/study record.

✔ Electronic messages and facsimiles should be printed, signed/dated, and filed in the site Regulatory Binder.

✔ Logs of procedures should exist.

✔ Records of calibration of study-required equipment, including temperature logs, should be kept and filed appropriately.

✔ Screening and recruitment logs (including computer-generated lists of potential study subjects) should be retained to demonstrate that inclusion/exclusion criteria were performed according to the Protocol.

✔ Site visit monitoring logs should be kept to document the purpose and frequency of the monitoring visit.

✔ Records of missing or unobtainable data required by the Protocol should be explained appropriately by a memo to the file, if applicable.

✔ If information must be added to a previous entry, it should be inserted and noted as a late entry or addendum at the end of the text in the medical chart. It should not be squeezed in between previously written notes.

✔ If data must be changed or clarified, the industry standard is to put a single line through the original entry, change the data, and initial and date the change.

✔ Any changes to the data should be evident in an audit trail. Explanations added to the progress notes may be required.

A source document is *always* a source document. It may seem a good idea to recopy a source document, instead of crossing out yet another entry and correcting it, *but* there is always the possibility of a transcription error. In addition, these and similar attempts to obliterate or destroy original data are *not* acceptable. To an auditor, these redactions may elicit suspicion. Is the motive fraud or neatness? Once redacted, the data is no longer a source document. *If it is not documented, it did not happen!*

E. Source Documentation Suggestions

The *Compliance Program Guidance Manual* used by the FDA to audit an investigative site is an excellent resource for source documentation. That, along with the industry standard, provides the rationale for the following documentation to support CRF data:

Notation that written, informed consent was obtained and that the consent form was dated and signed by the subject (or the subject's representative, if applicable) prior to the performance of any study-related procedure. It is generally a good idea to also note the time at which informed consent was obtained. This will confirm that study-related procedures, such as laboratory samples, were obtained after informed consent was obtained. If an Investigator's signature is required on the consent form, and the Investigator did not sign on the same date that the patient did, make sure the actual date that the Investigator signed the informed consent is used. Note in the source the reason for the later date. *Under no circumstances should a CRC enter patient's initials on the consent or enter the date for the patient.* The patient should perform these tasks by him/herself.

Record the date of entry into the study, the Sponsor's Protocol number, and the subject number.

The subject's diagnosis and current physical status prior to the initiation of any study-related procedures should be noted. Include details of medical history, checking the inclusion/exclusion criteria.

Record current medications, as well as medications discontinued within the past 30 days. Review the Protocol to determine if there are restricted or excluded medications and the wash-out period required by the Protocol. It is a good idea to ask potential subjects to bring their actual pill bottles to the screening visit. This way you can be sure the medication information being provided by the subject is accurate.

Document the name and/or number of the study drug dispensed, as well as the dosing information. Note the total amount of study drug dispensed at subsequent visits; include the amount of study drug returned by the subject. If there is a discrepancy, note the reason for it.

For example:

> *Patient #1234 did not return study drug dispensed on 4/10/04, inadvertently discarded empty bottle. Patient instructed on the importance of returning study drug, even if the bottle is empty.*

Patient #4562 missed two doses of study medication while on vacation. Patient instructed on the importance of taking the study drug according to the directions.

Patient #0001 did not return unused study medication dispensed on 5/8/04. Sponsor was contacted and gave approval to dispense additional medication. Patient will return unused study drug at the next visit. Patient instructed on the importance of returning unused medication at each visit.

Patient #6534 was screened for Protocol NA#0099 today. Informed consent was obtained prior to the initiation of any study-related procedures. The patient did not have any questions regarding the study or the study requirements. The patient understands his/her role as a study participant. The patient meets inclusion/exclusion criteria. Next visit scheduled for 6/10/04.

Document the dates and results of study-specific evaluations and procedures. Any deviations from the Protocol must be documented and reported to the Sponsor and the IRB.

Record all AEs and complaints noted by the subject during the study and for the appropriate time specified by the Protocol. Include the last dose of study drug taken by the patient and any medical intervention or action taken to treat the AE or complaint.

In study progress notes, record the subject's condition during and/or after treatment.

Note the final disposition of the subject and the subject's status at the time of study termination. This includes premature study termination. Make sure you note the reason for premature study termination. There is a difference between study drug termination and study termination. While a subject may be terminated from study drug treatment, the subject may not be terminated from the study. This is study- and Sponsor-specific.

The most frequent cause of disagreements between CRAs and CRCs is the adequacy of source documentation.

Notes to File

A common document many clinical sites are asked to create is a Note to File (NTF). Generally, a NTF is a memo and when used appropriately can be a positive practice.

A useful NTF includes the following:

- ✔ Identification of a problem that occurred during the conduct of the clinical trial
- ✔ Procedural change identified to correct the problem to prevent recurrence
- ✔ Institution of a procedural change

In the event of an inspection by the FDA or other regulatory agency, the inspector may still leave a citation for the initial problem, but the change in procedure mitigates the citation and provides the site with a strong response to the finding.

Many in the clinical trial community consider that an NTF is a panacea for all things that have not been done appropriately during the conduct of a clinical trial. Make a mistake? What are CRCs told, often by the CRA? Write an NTF, and put it in the Regulatory Binder and/or the subjects' source documents. This practice has become so ubiquitous that new CRAs and CRCs sometimes think NTFs are regulatory requirements, necessary to document and correct the problem to prevent it from recurring. This is a misconception. There is nothing in the FDA regulations or guidance documents requiring Sponsors and research sites to use an NTF.

Many research professionals think that an NTF is a corrective action. Many NTFs are quickly written without any regard to correcting the problem. Sometimes, the NTF is generated well after the deviation/problem has occurred and all is considered right with the pharmaceutical world, when this is not the case. In fact, the FDA recently reprimanded a Sponsor for "after-the-fact-memos."

In an FDA Warning Letter dated October 23, 2007 (www.fda.gov/foi/warning_letters/s6551c.htm), the FDA wrote: "Our investigation found the Sponsor failed to take any action except to generate numerous memos to file after all the subjects completed the study." The Warning Letter then noted at least 89 memos that were generated after a monitoring visit. Instead of writing an NTF, the Sponsor's time is better spent qualifying the site and training the study staff.

Documenting a mistake means absolutely nothing during an FDA inspection. Corrective action, and whether the corrective action was appropriate, should be what is documented. If a site does not have an effective quality system in place prior to the start of a clinical trial, especially subject enrollment, then the Sponsor, CRAs, PIs, and study staff will have an understanding of how the Protocol will be monitored and how discrepancies will be communicated and corrected. Sponsors cannot depend on post monitoring visit letters to demonstrate compliance in serious situations.

In my own auditing experience, I have noted that NTFs are frequently contentious issues between CRAs and the study staff. I have seen trivial NTFs placed in Regulatory Binders at the request of inexperienced CRAs. In addition, since they are asked to generate so many, some CRCs have developed a habit of writing NTFs instead of developing good recordkeeping practices, or, in some cases in place of having SOPs. All an NTF accomplishes is documenting poor performance, and ineffective work rarely impresses the FDA.

Conducting clinical trials according to all the regulations and guidelines is hard work and requires professional cooperation to quickly address queries and genuine findings that need correcting. Once an NTF is written and becomes a study document, it cannot be retracted. The result is a lose-lose situation for everyone involved in the study. These NTFs are a road map for any inspector, showing all the mistakes made during the conduct of the Protocol. Perhaps a better solution is to develop a quality system of SOPs from the beginning. These SOPs should include training on the Protocol, documenting the informed consent process, delegation of authority tasks, storage of the investigational product, how data corrections are made, and how problems are identified and corrected. These SOPs should be provided to all study staff so there is consistency during the clinical trial. Sites should document the corrective action and keep NTFs few and far between.

According to Carl Anderson's, Senior Consultant for Biologics Consulting Group, Note to Self: No More Notes to File!

F. Meeting the Requirements of Source Documentation

✔ Study-specific labels attached to progress notes;

✔ Protocol-specific flow sheets;

✔ Protocol-specific checklists; and

✔ Protocol-specific templates created by the site or in some instances the Sponsor, to collect the data required by the CRF.

A discussion between the Sponsor and/or the CRO/SMO concerning their expectations regarding source documentation prior to the initiation of the study is essential. This will avoid problems in the future. It is a good idea to obtain written requests for any requirements that deviated from your site's SOPs. In advance, evaluate the source documentation requirements, and evaluate the extent to which you can comply. Do not hesitate to negotiate what is acceptable to all parties concerned. Educate the medical record department about the importance of research records.

Document any violations and/or deviations from procedures specified by the Protocol and the reason. This represents changes made to the Protocol that have not been approved by the Sponsor or the IRB. Since they may affect risk to the research subject and will impact the integrity of the data, violations and/or deviations play an important part in Warning Letters issued by the FDA.

All allied health professionals involved in the conduct of clinical research are responsible for conducting research ethically. The complete, accurate, and thorough documentation of the research subject's participation in the Protocol enables the research site to demonstrate that the requirements for GCP were fulfilled during the conduct of the research study.

G. Data Clarification and Adverse Event Reporting

Adverse Events

ICH guidelines define an AE as:

> Any untoward medical occurrence in a patient or clinical investigation subject administered a pharmaceutical product and which does not necessarily have a causal relationship with this treatment. An AE can therefore be any unfavorable or unintended sign, which

includes abnormal laboratory results, symptom, or disease temporally associated with the use of a medicinal (Investigational) product.

To prove to regulatory agencies that they are safe and effective, drugs undergo extensive testing. AEs are one aspect of this safety evaluation, and it is important that any AEs that occur in a study are reported accurately and promptly.

AEs must be in *appropriate* medical terminology with sufficient information to ensure that the occurrence is accurately recorded so that it can easily be matched against a coding dictionary such as MedDRA, COSTATR, WHOART, or ICD9.

When an AE is recorded, the terms used must be unambiguous, in acceptable English (although Latin terms can be used), and *with no spelling errors*.

Most of the examples used in this chapter have been recorded from actual clinical trials and are used to illustrate problems encountered by Data Management when recording AEs.

Common Problems

Two Conditions Reported as One Adverse Event

- ✔ Anxious and insomnia
- ✔ Rash and fatigue
- ✔ Dizziness and nausea
- ✔ Muscle ache and back pain
- ✔ Nausea and asthenia
- ✔ Leucocytosis and fever
- ✔ Disorientation/agitation

The conditions noted are *different* AEs and cannot be coded together. These conditions must be separated into two individual AEs. For example: Anxious will be mapped to a dictionary term of anxiety, whereas insomnia will be mapped to insomnia. In the case of dizziness and nausea, dizziness will be mapped to a dictionary term of dizziness and body system Nervous System, but nausea will be mapped to a body system Digestive System. Nausea and vomiting must be split into two AEs if the MedDRA dictionary is being used for coding.

Medical Abbreviations

The use of medical abbreviations must be done with care. Refer to a standard reference book, such as *Medical Abbreviations*, 8th Edition (Neil M. Davis). For example:

✔ "Worsening RA" could mean worsening rales or worsening rheumatoid arthritis.

✔ "Worsening of AP" may denote worsening acute pancreatitis, worsening appendicitis, or worsening arterial pressure.

✔ "Increased DM" can be taken to mean increased dermatomyositis, increased diabetes mellitus, or increased diastolic murmur.

✔ "CHF," as well as being the medical abbreviation of chronic heart failure, can also be Crimean hemorrhagic fever or congestive heart failure.

✔ "C.O.L.D." means chronic obstructive lung disease not coryza (common cold).

✔ "LAH" refers to either left anterior hemiblock or left atrial hypertrophy.

✔ "CM" could mean common migraine, continuous murmur, or chondromalacia.

Truncated Words

AE text should not be shortened.

✔ "FR left ankle" may be assumed to be a fracture of the left ankle, but the abbreviation for fracture is incorrect and should be FS or #. For clarity it would be preferable to use the word FRACTURE.

✔ "FR" is a medical abbreviation for "fluid restriction" and "factional reabsorption," as well as father.

✔ Pleurit could have many possible interpretations: pleuritic pain, pleuritis, etc.

Laboratory Data

In the case of changes in biochemistry of the blood or in alterations in hematology parameters, it must be specified if there was a measured increase or decrease:

✔ "Calcium"   increased calcium or decreased calcium?

✔ "LFTs"   decreased liver enzymes or increased LFTs?

✔ "Hg"   elevated hemoglobin or decreased hemoglobin?

✔ "↓ Platelets"   reduced platelets

Symptom versus Medical Diagnosis

Provide a diagnosis instead of a list of symptoms.

✔ "Upper respiratory tract infection" rather than "runny nose," "sore throat," "hoarseness," "sinus problem," "fever," etc.

✔ "Diarrhea" is preferred to the symptoms of "loose liquid stools," "increased frequency," and "abdominal pain."

✔ "Cold" could refer to an upper respiratory chest infection or a feeling of being cold; the term should be made specific to the problem reported.

Modifiers

Some medical terms need additional information to more completely describe the AE being reported. For example:

✔ "Cirrhosis"   can pertain to brain, kidney, liver, lung, malarial, ovarian, pancreas, spleen, or stomach

✔ "Caries"   can refer to either bone or tooth

✔ "Amputation"   can be surgical or traumatic

✔ "Abortion"   can be therapeutic or spontaneous

✔ "Fibrocystic Disease" can be fibrocystic breast disease or cystic fibrosis

✔ "Herpes"   can be simplex or zoster

✔ "Kaposi's"   can refer to Kaposi's disease, Kaposi's sarcoma, or varicelliform eruption

✔ "Stiffness"   can describe muscles or joints

✔ "Ulcer"   can refer to gastric, stomach, duodenal, skin, corneal, or decubitis

✔ "Cramps"   can refer to muscle or abdominal

✔ "Edema"   can be dependent, ankle, tongue, pharynx, face, peripheral, etc.

✔ "Hemorrhage"   unless describing a generalized hemorrhage, the site of the hemorrhage should be recorded: gastrointestinal hemorrhage, gum hemorrhage, gastric hemorrhage, etc.

✔ "Reflux"   can be gastrointestinal or kidney

✔ "Hernia"   can be umbilical, inguinal, or hiatal

✔ "Incontinence"   can be urinary, fecal, or stress

Infections
Record either the site of the infection or the organism involved:

   ✔ In the case of a respiratory tract infection, note whether it is an upper or lower respiratory chest infection.

   ✔ Eye infections can be of several types and should be specified: conjunctivitis, iritis, keratitis, retinitis, scleritis, uveitis, or kearatonconjunctivitis.

   ✔ Ear infections can be divided into otitis media, otitis externa, otitis interna, etc., depending on the site.

Sore
The word "sore" means either a lesion or a feeling of soreness.

Language
Care should be given to the meaning of the word used on the CRF, as the entry may not be obvious to the person later entering the database.

"Angina" is defined in medical dictionaries as pain. Commonly, angina is taken to mean angina pectoris, but the term could or should be queried to ensure that this is the correct AE.

In France, "angina" is used for tonsillitis, and staff has queried French sites to ensure that a tonsillectomy is the correct treatment for angina. In Europe, "hypotonia" and "hypertonia" are commonly used terms for hypotension and hypertension. Elsewhere, however, standard medical dictionaries use these terms to mean decreased or increased tension in any part of the body (for example, muscle hypotonia, arterial wall hypertonia, or oscular hypertonia). The meaning of the term used should be investigated to ensure the correct term is being used for the condition being reported.

Pain
Pain terms should specify a site where the pain is located. The use of the word "pain" alone is not enough information to allow for the proper coding of the AE.

"Chest pain" can be either muscle or cardiac pain, and the type should be specified.

Rashes
When reporting a rash, be sure to include not only the type of rash, i.e., macular rash or erythematous rash, but also the location of the rash. This information may be important, especially in a dermatology study or in a study where the study medication being used is known to possibly cause a rash.

Nonsense Words
Some AEs reported using nonmedical words and phrases may be queried. The following words have actually been used when reporting an AE:

- ✔ "Eruptions"
- ✔ "Increase in peptic symptoms"
- ✔ "Heat waves"
- ✔ "Root fracture"
- ✔ "Relaxed bowels"
- ✔ "GIT gases"
- ✔ "Elevation"
- ✔ "Blushing groin"
- ✔ "Gastric juice"
- ✔ "Wants to stop smoking"
- ✔ "Erection"
- ✔ "Temperature"
- ✔ "Erections disappeared"
- ✔ "Patient complains of 'funny head'"
- ✔ "Urinalysis pH9"
- ✔ "Farsightedness"
- ✔ "Fogginess"
- ✔ "Odd feeling in head"
- ✔ "Elbow twist"
- ✔ "Urine color pink"
- ✔ "Pacing"
- ✔ "Desaturation"
- ✔ "Large occult blood"
- ✔ "Left shin in differential"
- ✔ "Broken ribbon"
- ✔ "Nervosity"
- ✔ "She feels like she has a cloud in her head"
- ✔ "Patient 100% noncompliant: medication eaten by her dog on return from surgery: dog slept for 3 days and made a full recovery with sequelae"
- ✔ "Increase in brightness of vision"

✔ "Unusually enhanced alcoholic effect"

✔ "Penile bend"

✔ "Hematological failure"

✔ "Speech"

✔ "Jar of the left ear"

✔ "Frozen"

✔ "Goat attack"

✔ "Jumping Heart"

✔ "Eye injury—attacked by bird"

✔ "Adenoid Vegetation"

H. Queries
The Data Clarification Process

For many Study Coordinators, the Data Clarification Process is one of the most troubling and time-consuming components of conducting clinical research projects.

Study Coordinators often believe that the number of queries generated during a clinical trial is a negative reflection of their work. In some instances this may be true but not in the majority of instances. Queries are considered by most CRCs as a dreaded event. For the most part, queries are generated for many reasons, such as:

✔ Amendments to the protocol

✔ Changes in CRF design

✔ Statistical program changes

✔ Clarification regarding information contained on the CRF

✔ Providing incomplete data on a CRF

✔ Providing too much information

✔ Spelling errors

The query or data process for a clinical trial begins when the Protocol and CRFs are designed and ends when all queries have been resolved and the database is locked in preparation for FDA submission. The process may vary from Sponsor to Sponsor and from project to project. However, the resolution of these queries is an intricate part of the clinical trial and is a critical component to the submission of the data collected during the clinical trial for presentation to the FDA.

The Data Process from Start to Finish

In order to understand the data process resulting in the generation of queries it is important to know exactly how the process works. The process may vary from project to project and from Sponsor to Sponsor, however it still results in the generation of queries. In addition, there is generally a specific time specified by the Sponsor to resolve these queries.

The following timeline is an example of how the data process typically works:

PROTOCOL AND CASE REPORT FORM RECEIVED
↓
DATABASE DESIGNED AND TESTED
↓
DATA REVIEW CONVENTIONS CREATED
↓
ELECTRONIC DATA CHECKS PROGRAMMED
↓
INVESTIGATOR MEETING
↓
DATA COLLECTED AND SENT TO THE SPONSOR
↓
COLLECTED DATA IS ENTERED
↓
ELECTRONIC DATA CHECKS PERFORMED
↓
AUTOENCODING TO STANDARD DICTIONARIES
↓
FAILED DATA CHECKS AND FAILED AUTOENCODING OUTPUT
↓
MANUAL AND ELECTRONIC REVIEW OF THE DATA
↓
GENERATION OF QUERIES
↓
QUERIES RETURNED
↓
DATA UPDATED
↓

CHECKS AND AUTOENCODING RERUN
QUERIES GENERATED
↓
DATA UPDATED AND CLEAN
↓
DATABASE IS LOCKED

I. Identifying Data Problems

Report forms and routine monitoring visits may reduce the number of data problems that could be resolved during the completion of the CRF.

Most Common Data Offenses

1. Providing incomplete data
2. Providing too much data
3. Misspelling
4. Providing ambiguous data

Providing Incomplete Data

✔ Frequently provides AE and concomitant medication data without the required supporting information

✔ Leaves required boxes on the CRF pages unchecked

✔ Indicates procedures on the CRF as Not Done (ND) when a review of the source documents indicate the procedures captured in the source documentation have actually been performed

How to Work with Incomplete Data

✔ Look for questions that have not been answered.

✔ Explain data that is missing, that is ND.

✔ If appropriate, cross out, date, and initial CRF pages that will not be completed and explain the reason this information is not available.

✔ Look for boxes that are not checked.

✔ Verify the information contained in the source documents is consistent with the information recorded on the CRF pages.

✔ Provide start and stop dates for AEs—indicate if they are ongoing or resolved. Document if treatment was given for verifying the treatment and if the dose if appropriate, recorded according to the Sponsor's requirements.

Providing Too Much Data

- ✔ Provides too much information for a single question

- ✔ Combines AEs or medication on one line

- ✔ Provides Investigator comments; while frequently providing extra information, these comments should be provided in a completely different place on the CRF

How to Work with Too Much Data

- ✔ Scrutinize the source documentation, especially the medical history, AEs, and medication pages for consistency.

- ✔ Verify AEs, medications, medical history, and prior surgical procedures are recorded on a separate line of specific CRF page.

- ✔ Look for data on the CRF pages that do not belong on that specific page.

- ✔ Cross-check AE pages with the medical history, current medical conditions, and medication pages to verify the information on the CRF is accurate and complete.

- ✔ Verify there are no AEs recorded that have been erroneously reported.

- ✔ Verify scheduled surgery has not been listed as an AE.

- ✔ Scrutinize the medication page of the CRF to ensure the start date of the medication that is started at the time of the AE has been noted.

- ✔ Verify medical conditions documented at the beginning of the study on the medical history CRF page have actually worsened since the start of the subject's participation in the study.

Misspelling

- ✔ Places extra letters haphazardly

- ✔ Frequently spells words wrong

- ✔ Frequently uses symbols such as ⇕; +; ≤; ≥; ± instead of proper terms

- ✔ Writes with moderate to severe illegibility, necessitating inquiry and clarifications

How to Work with Misspelling

- ✔ Verify commonly misspelled words such as AEs and medications to ensure they are spelled correctly.

- ✔ Clarify data that is illegible before the best person to decipher it, the author, leaves.

✔ Scrutinize abbreviations to ensure the CRF guidelines allow for the use of abbreviations—if it is not a common abbreviation, it must be defined.

Providing Ambiguous Data

✔ Frequently provides symptoms rather than diagnosis

✔ Uses words like "fell," "pain," and "accident" to describe events that need further clarification

✔ Supplies data requiring further clarification, i.e., "Ear Infection"—Is it Otitis Interna, Otitis Media, or Otitis Externia? Herpes—Simplex or Zoster? Diabetes —Mellitus or Insipidus?

✔ Uses the word "prophylaxis" without a medical reason

How to Work with Ambiguous Data

✔ Look for terms that will need clarification: e.g., "fall," "pain," "accident," and "infection," "antibiotic," or "cold."

✔ Cross-check AE CRF pages with the concomitant medications and medical history pages to find unreported AEs.

✔ Know what medical terms can be coded.

✔ Verify the AEs reported are valid.

✔ Verify start and stop dates for AEs ("unknown" is not acceptable except on very rare occasions).

✔ Clarify the medical reason a concomitant medication is being taken prophylaxis, i.e., for vitamins, health supplement, or baby aspirin (cardiac prophylaxis)

The objectives of completing the CRFs appropriately are to:

✔ Increase the quality of the data recorded

✔ Increase the knowledge of the site's staff

✔ Decrease the number of queries

✔ Decrease stress for Investigator, coordinators, monitors, and data managers

✔ Decrease late state project timelines

✔ Decrease the amount of work for the site's staff

✔ Decrease project overruns

✔ Enable safer drugs to be brought to market faster

VII. Obtaining Informed Consent and Assent Approval

A. Obtaining Informed Consent

The law requires obtaining informed consent from each potential subject before that subject may participate in a clinical study or be screened for the study with clinical or laboratory procedures not normally carried out on similar subjects. The Code of Federal Regulations (21 CFR, Part 50, Subpart B) explains the details of informed consent.

The design and construction of an Informed consent form is the responsibility of the PI, but the Sponsor usually provides guidance in preparing the document and, possibly, the completed sample documents. In addition, the informed consent form must be reviewed and approved by the IRB at each participating institution *before* it can be used.

Informed consent is not just a document; it is a process. In order to assure that a subject adequately understands the study, many sites use documentation forms that are completed by the person obtaining consent and that may consist of questions and scored answers that the subject has given. The person obtaining the consent signs and dates these forms, which are included in the subject's research file.

One of the most important responsibilities of the CRC is to make sure that every potential subject (or that a subject's duly authorized representative) reads, understands, and signs an informed consent form before participating in a study.

Furthermore, the CRC must be sure that all signatures, dates, and other required information have been obtained. The CRC can reassure the potential subject there is nothing wrong with asking the CRC to explain the clinical trial in everyday, layperson's language. It is also important for the CRC to ensure a potential subject is able to understand a consent form written in English. If this is not the case, the Sponsor can and should provide study-related documents such as the informed consent, study-specific questionnaires, and so on in the potential subject's primary language. There are, however, some studies that include only English-speaking subjects. In those cases, the subject should not participate in those studies if he/she is not able to understand the English-language documents. There are exceptions to this, however, and these exceptions may be granted by the Sponsor and approved by the IRB, if applicable.

For those clinical trials open to different foreign languages, all aspects of the clinical trial should be presented to a subject in any language that will enable the subject to make an informed decision when consenting to participate in a clinical trial.

According to CenterWatch, for nearly 8 million volunteers who participate in government and pharmaceutical industry-sponsored clinical trials each year in the United States alone, the informed consent process is a rite of passage. When the volunteer consents to participate in a clinical trial, as noted previously, it is important for the potential subject to acknowledge understanding all aspects of the clinical trial, as well as the risks involved, in order to make an informed decision to participate in the clinical trial. While the CRC may be part of the informed consent process, it is ultimately the PI's responsibility to ensure a potential subject completely understands everything contained in the informed consent document. The PI will provide additional time for the potential subject to review the informed consent document, take it home, and discuss participation with family members, which may raise important questions regarding the potential subject's participation in the clinical trial.

A potential subject should also understand the main reason for participating in a clinical trial is for the advancement of science not to obtain treatment for a disease.

It is important for the potential subject to be informed that the person conducting the study has the responsibility to follow the clinical trial Protocol exactly as it is written and approved by the IRB.

The informed consent form is designed to give the subject or legal representative *easy-to-understand information* regarding the following aspects of the study:

- ✔ general design and purpose of the study;
- ✔ total length of the study;
- ✔ number of visits required for the study;
- ✔ total number of subjects in the study and number at the subject's particular site;
- ✔ benefits of the study treatment;

- ✔ risks of the study treatment;

- ✔ side effects associated with the study treatment;

- ✔ specified procedures unique to the study and risks involved;

- ✔ that the subject may receive a placebo and not active treatment (if applicable);

- ✔ alternative therapies that the subject may be offered;

- ✔ right of the subject to withdraw with no penalty;

- ✔ whom to contact 24 hours a day in case of questions or emergencies;

- ✔ confidentiality of subject records;

- ✔ costs and compensation; and

- ✔ compensation or medical treatments available for any research-related injury.

During the informed consent process, the potential subject may ask the following questions about the clinical trial to confirm his/her understanding of the written informed consent document. The person obtaining the consent should also question the potential subject to assure that there is a good level of understanding.

- ✔ What is the main purpose of the study?

- ✔ Why is this study important to me?

- ✔ What are the chances that this drug will work?

- ✔ What kinds of risks are involved?

- ✔ How much time from my daily schedule will this take?

- ✔ Does the study involve a placebo or a treatment already available?

While these elements are in the informed consent document, in many instances, potential subjects want to ensure they also understand their responsibilities in participating in a clinical trial.

Potential volunteers care about the following:

- ✔ What kinds of tests will be done?

- ✔ Will the tests hurt?

- ✔ How much blood will be taken (tubes not approximate amounts, tablespoon, etc.), as well as the frequency of the blood sample collection, if blood samples are required for the clinical trial?

- ✔ How will the tests in the clinical trial compare to tests conducted outside of the clinical trial?

- ✔ Would the potential subject be able to see his/her own physician?

✔ Would the potential subject be able to take regularly prescribed medications while participating in the clinical trial?

✔ How would any side effects experienced during the clinical trial participation be treated?.

In 2002, CenterWatch conducted a survey of nearly 1,600 clinical trial volunteers regarding ways the informed consent process is working and where it is breaking down. The survey showed:

✔ The vast majority of potential study volunteers claim to understand their responsibility in participating in a clinical trial, including their ability to withdraw at any time. A total of 69 percent indicated they understood this information, and 11 percent indicated they did not understand this information.

✔ A high percentage of volunteers indicated they did not fully understand all of the risks involved with participation in the clinical trial. Seventy percent understood there were additional risks and discomforts, while 30 percent were not sure.

✔ A significant number of potential study subjects, based upon the information noted above, are not reading the informed consent form.

There appears to be a wide variability among potential study volunteers when it comes to asking a lot of questions and to being engaged through a discussion of a Protocol-specific clinical trial informed consent form. In the CenterWatch survey previously noted, 70 percent of respondents to the survey indicated they didn't even know what questions to ask the study staff.

Perhaps one reason a high number of study subjects drop out of a clinical trial is because many subjects do not fully understand what they are consenting to from the beginning. It is in the potential study subject's best interest, as well as the site's, to find out as much as possible about the potential study subject's comprehension before the actual informed consent document is signed. The CenterWatch study noted 84 percent of the potential subjects surveyed indicated their questions had been answered to their satisfaction, while 16 percent were not sure. Approximately 60 percent of the potential subjects surveyed were aware they could contact someone other than the study staff if they had questions about their rights, while 40 percent were not sure they could contact someone other than the study staff regarding their rights.

The FDA guidelines indicate that potential study volunteers should fully understand the risks of the test article being researched. While you do not want to influence the potential subject regarding the risks, it is important to be objective so that the potential subject can understand the information contained in the informed consent document.

While the test article may make the potential study subject feel better, and the study office visits may seem like any other visit to a doctor's office, subjects need to be reminded they are volunteering for a clinical trial, whose main purpose is to collect data not to treat illness.

The rationale and basic content of informed consent have been set forth by FDA regulations. These regulations are described in the CFR, which may be obtained from the FDA (see Appendix I for contact information). While informed consent has traditionally been obtained by providing each subject with a written description of the elements of the study, some organizations are using novel approaches to educate prospective subjects. One of the most intriguing methods involves the presentation of the informed consent information in a video format, in conjunction with the written document. This approach is particularly useful for demonstrating difficult-to-explain procedures (such as cardiac catheterization, a novel surgical technique, and how to complete a patient diary) and gives the subject a visual opportunity to assess the risks and benefits associated with the study.

B. Obtaining Institutional Review Board Approvals

An IRB has at least five members with a diverse background of experience. The diversity of the IRB members' backgrounds will ensure cultural, educational, and racial diversity reflecting that of the local community. Members may include physicians, nurses, clergy, social workers, lawyers, and ethics experts. This enables the IRB to make an assessment of the validity of the study objectives. The Code of Federal Regulations (21 CFR) Part 56 reviews the regulatory considerations associated with IRBs.

Approval of a Protocol by the IRB is required in the following three situations. In each case, proper documentation for the approval is required.

Initial IRB Approval. Generally, initial review and approval by the IRB of the Protocol, the Investigator, subinvestigators, the site(s), and the study site's informed consent form and advertisement (if applicable) is required before enrollment can begin

Until the Investigator receives written IRB approval, no subject can undergo any procedures for the purpose of determining eligibility for the study.

Protocol Amendment IRB Approval. Should an amendment to the Protocol become advisable, in most cases, IRB approval must be received before the amendment can be implemented. In emergency situations, the amendment may be implemented first and the IRB notified within 10 days.

Continuing IRB Approval. Continuing IRB approval must be obtained for studies that last for more than one year or other specified period. This will consist of documentation of the IRB's annual review and continuing approval of the Protocol. The frequency of reporting the progress of a clinical trial varies from IRB to IRB. Be sure to know the reporting requirements for the IRB used for each Protocol.

Continuing IRB approval is obtained minimally on the annual anniversary date of the original approval and yearly thereafter, or as specified by the IRB, for as long as the study continues. The site may also be audited by the IRB to ensure the study is being conducted properly. If the IRB requires a fee, a note describing this fee (known as the "IRB Fee Letter") should not be included in the Study File.

C. Reviewing the Protocol and Obtaining Signatures

Each clinical study must have a written Protocol, which is the document that gives specific instructions for the conduct of the study. Approval of the Protocol by the IRB must be obtained *before* any subjects are allowed to participate or are requested formally to consent to participate in the investigation.

In addition, the PI must submit significant changes or amendments to the Protocol to the IRB if such a change increases the risk to subjects or adversely affects the validity of the investigation or the rights of the subjects. The Investigator must obtain approval by the IRB before such change or deviation is implemented. When the change is made to eliminate or reduce the risk to subjects, it may be implemented before the review or approval by the IRB. In these instances, the Investigator is required to notify the IRB, in writing, of the change within 10 days after implementation.

All changes or revisions to the Protocol, and the reasons for those changes, must be documented, dated, and maintained with the Protocol.

Before the site initiation visit with the Sponsor, the Investigator and CRCs must read the Protocol. They should highlight important topics and identify any questions that need clarification by the Sponsor or CRO/SMO.

D. HIPAA Regulations and Clinical Research

On April 14, 2003, the HIPAA regulations went into effect as a federal law. HIPAA stands for the Health Insurance Portability and Accountability Act of 1996. HIPAA is a privacy rule providing federal protection for the privacy of protected health information. HIPAA also protects against the misuse of individually identifiable health information.

How HIPAA Will Affect Clinical Research

- ✔ Research subjects must sign a document that allows access to their protected health information necessary for the subject to participate in a clinical trial. Research sites will implement one of the following policies:

    1. Some IRBs will use the Sponsor's HIPAA authorization form as a stand-alone document.

    2. Some IRBs will incorporate the required HIPAA language into the informed consent form.

- ✔ Current subjects in an active clinical trial who have already signed an informed consent to participate in the active clinical trial were grandfathered into the regulation and did not need to sign a revised informed consent or authorization form, unless directed by the research site's local IRB.

- ✔ Research subjects who signed an informed consent document on or after April 14, 2003, must sign the revised informed consent document or an authorization HIPAA form to allow the Sponsor's representative access to their protected health information.

- ✔ Clinical trials that had not been initiated on or after April 14, 2003, and all new clinical trials will have verbiage in their contracts confirming they will only enroll subjects in clinical trials willing to sign the authorization.

✔ HIPPAA will have an impact on research site selection and the prescreening of potential subject charts.

HIPAA Required Elements for Authorization

A HIPAA authorization form must contain the following required elements

✔ description of the information to be used or disclosed in a specific and meaningful fashion;

✔ identification of the person(s) authorized to make the requested use or disclosure;

✔ identification of the person(s) to whom the covered entity may make the requested use or disclosure;

✔ description of the purpose or the use or disclosure;

✔ expiration date or event;

✔ signature of the individual and date (personal representative is allowed if description of representative's authority to act for the individual is provided)

✔ statement of the individual's right to revoke the authorization and that revocation must be in writing;

✔ statement of consequences of the individual's refusal to sign the authorization;

✔ statement of the potential for information to be redisclosed by the recipient and thus no longer protected by this subpart;

✔ statement of the individual's agreement to denial of access to personal health information created or obtained for research purposes while the clinical trial is in process;

✔ authorization must be in lay language; and

✔ a copy of the signed authorization must be provided to the individual.

E. Clinical Research: Study Assent in Adolescents/Children

Adult patients have the right to informed consent, and it is now recognized that adolescents and children have a similar right to have this same study information explained to them in suitable language. They should be able to understand the nature and impact of what treatments they may receive if they participate in a study.

However, legally, children cannot provide informed consent. The parents or legal guardians must be responsible for the child's participation in a clinical study. IRBs consider children to be a vulnerable subgroup and may require special protections to assure that studies are conducted ethically.

Therefore, physicians and parents should not exclude adolescents and children from the decision making process but provide an opportunity for them to understand the risks and benefits of treatment and be informed of alternative treatments, including the risks and benefits of no treatment.

In medical matters, the ultimate treatment decision will be made by physicians and parents who are focused on the best interests of the child. These adults have an ethical and legal obligation to provide the best competent medical care. Although investigators may receive a parent's approval on the informed consent form, they should plan how to address dissent from the child. Legally the physician can proceed but what is the effect on the child's concerns and cooperation?

It is suggested that an informed assent document include:

1. Information written on a level appropriate to the development of the adolescent/child

2. Details of the nature of the disease, or condition

3. Which tests and treatments to expect with details on risks and benefits, including the consequences of no treatment

4. A real opportunity for the adolescent/child to ask questions and clarifications of the assent document

Physicians and parents should be prepared for adolescents/children to refuse assent for treatment, and the parents and physician must then weigh the medical consequences against the wishes of the adolescent/child.

IRBs usually have standard language templates for parental permission and patient assent forms and procedures. These templates vary depending on patient age, therapeutic area, study design, risks and benefits to the patient, and state regulations concerning care and treatment of adolescents and children.

Some IRBs will prepare two documents: an informed consent for the parents to review and sign, and a separate assent form with simpler language for the child.

Finally, in the case of very young children unaccustomed to signing documents, some IRBs will provide a space for an independent third party (patient advocate) to verify by signature that the study was explained to the child and the assent of the child was obtained.

On some occasions, the IRB may determine that a child's assent may not be necessary for proceeding with the trial. This situation would depend on the prospect of a clear direct benefit of the treatment or procedure to the child.

VIII. Pertinent Forms and Study Records

A. The Test Article Inventory System

The Test Article Inventory System will dictate where test articles are to be stored and who will keep track of the amount of test articles received, dispensed, and returned to the Sponsor. The inventory system must ensure that:

✔ adequate supplies are always on hand;

✔ test articles are stored securely and in the proper environment (e.g., the refrigerator), including controlled substances;

✔ the Drug Accountability Record is properly maintained;

✔ there is agreement between the number of test articles received versus the number of test articles dispensed (as recorded on the Drug Accountability Record and CRFs versus the number of test articles on hand;

✔ the dispensing record and the CRFs agree concerning the identification of subjects receiving the test article;

✔ shipping/packing forms are properly addressed according to Sponsor instructions;

✔ the test articles have not expired or have not been recalled by the Sponsor; and

✔ all test articles returned by subjects are accurately counted and recorded.

The CRA will need access to the test article storage area during site visits to verify the status of the test article supply. While some site-specific SOPs may not allow CRAs into the drug storage area due to confidentiality issues, the CRA must be able to document that the test article is being stored according to the specific Protocol requirements.

B. The Drug Accountability Record

The PI or designee (typically the CRC) is responsible for dispensing and accounting for the test articles and for exercising GCP guidelines in monitoring these supplies. The dispensing and return of test articles must be entered promptly on the Drug Accountability Record. The Sponsor or CRO/SMO should supply this form.

Under no circumstances should the PI supply test articles to other investigators, study sites, or non-study patients, nor should he/she allow the test articles to be used in a manner other than as directed by the Protocol.

Test articles returned by a subject must be entered on the Drug Accountability Record and set aside for return to the Sponsor. *They must not be redispensed to anyone—not even to the same subject. Note: Study drug returned must be stored separately from study drug not yet dispensed*

At the termination of the study, or at the request of the Sponsor or CRO/SMO, the CRA will collect all remaining supplies, and the final Drug Accountability Record will be completed. These will then be delivered to the Sponsor. A copy of the Drug Accountability Record should be retained in the Study File. All manifests documenting shipments of test articles should be retained as well, along with copies of a returned goods form, if provided.

In some instances, the Sponsor will request the test article to be destroyed on site. A copy of your site's SOPs for the destruction of test articles at your site will need to be provided to the Sponsor prior to the destruction of any test article. Once the test article is destroyed, a Certificate of Destruction will need to be completed, documenting exactly what was destroyed, and provided to the Sponsor.

During site visits, the CRA will typically be required to make a 100 percent source document verification of all dispensing and return data that appear on the Drug Accountability Record.

C. Paper Case Report Forms

CRFs provide for the orderly transfer of data from the study site to the CRO/SMO or Sponsor. CRFs are preprinted pages that allow the Investigator or CRC to write in appropriate data regarding demography, efficacy, safety, medication use, and other aspects of the study. Therefore, it is of the utmost importance that data are entered properly and accurately on the CRF. Currently, at many sites there are data coordinators completing CRFs from the same documentation. These data coordinators work closely with the CRC in the completion of the CRFs.

The following guidelines should be followed when completing CRFs:

- ✔ All entries should be completed legibly using a *black* ballpoint pen or a typewriter.
- ✔ Only acceptable medical terminology and standard abbreviations should be used.
- ✔ Care should be taken not to write on any other forms placed on top of the CRF (written impressions will transfer to all copies of the carbonless forms underneath).

✔ Time should be entered as military time (a conversion chart is provided in Appendix III, Part A).

✔ Numbers should be used to indicate dates (e.g., 10-01-02, not Oct. 1, 2002), unless otherwise specified.

✔ When completing the CRF and other documents pertaining to the study, there must be a response to every question so that the study data is complete for later entry into the Sponsor's database. Blank spaces, question marks, or zeros should not be used for unknown quantities. Instead, in cases where the data requested are unavailable, the following abbreviations can be used:

N/Av—not available. This abbreviation is used when the data are not available because they are not retrievable, the subject cannot remember, or the data were lost.

N/A—not applicable. This should be used for data that do not apply to the subject. For example, if the CRF calls for the date of the last pelvic examination and the subject is a man, "N/A" should be entered.

N/D—not done. This is entered when the data were not obtained. For example, if a vital sign such as blood pressure was requested but was not measured, enter "N/D."

Note: Sponsors may provide the site with a list of acceptable, study-specific abbreviations.

✔ Each item should be answered or checked individually rather than by using vertical lines or "ditto" marks to indicate a series of identical answers. The CRA needs to verify that the item was addressed.

Any discrepancies or missing data noted by the CRC or the CRA during site visits should be resolved before the data are forwarded to the CRO/SMO or Sponsor. A memo to file may be required to explain missing data or discrepancies, as well as deviations from Protocol.

Corrections should be made in the following manner:

✔ The original entry should be crossed out with a single line drawn through the error so it remains legible (not erased, written over, or covered up by correction fluid).

✔ The correction should be entered in ink and initialed and dated by the person making the correction.

Only the PI or the designee listed on the Authorized Representative Signature Record (Site Signature Log) may enter corrections on original CRFs.

The CRA is responsible for inspecting every page of data before the CRFs are sent to the Sponsor or CRO/SMO. This inspection generally consists of a complete audit of all laboratory test values, the signed informed consent forms, and critical nonlaboratory data (e.g., inclusion and exclusion criteria) against the source documents. In addition, a spot-check of at least 20 percent of all other data is typically performed. The CRA will also check for legibility, completeness, and consistency.

Before a review of the CRFs is conducted, the CRC should be sure that all forms are available, completed, and signed for the CRA's inspection within two weeks of study subject contact and provide explanations for missing data (e.g., delayed laboratory reports).

The CRC is responsible for making sure that all CRFs have been dated and signed by either the PI or an associate named on Form FDA 1572. If an associate signs CRFs, the Investigator must provide signed documentation that affirms his/her review and approval of the CRFs before their release to the CRO/SMO or Sponsor. The final signature of the Investigator on the CRF is generally done when all study inquiries and/or outstanding issues have been resolved. Your CRA will let you know when the Investigator can sign the final CRF signature page.

D. Authorized Representative Signature Record (Site Signature Log)

The Authorized Representative Signature Record is maintained at each clinical study site to document the full name, handwritten signature, and initials of the PI and the representatives who are authorized to complete and/or make changes to the CRFs. A copy of this document should be maintained in the on-site investigator Study File.

If newly authorized representatives are assigned during the study, a new Authorized Representative Signature Record will be initiated for those signatures. This information should also be forwarded to the Sponsor.

E. The Adverse Experience Form

An adverse experience can be broadly defined as a medical complaint, change, or possible side effect of any degree of severity that may or may not be attributed to the test article. The reporting of adverse experiences is an extremely important part of conducting a clinical study, and the CRC plays a vital role in the proper and timely reporting of adverse experiences and their follow-ups.

The Adverse Experience Form included in the CRF packet provided by the Sponsor is used to record events that the investigator regards as adverse experiences (see Appendix II, Form 7). The Investigator has the final decision regarding what is to be reported on the Adverse Experience Form, but the CRA may question the Investigator about including unreported complaints found in the source documents or reported in other documents included in the CRF. If there is a question regarding where any study subject information is to be reported, the CRA should be contacted.

Some Sponsors list concomitant medications on Adverse Experience Forms because the event may be related to the concomitant medication and not the test drug.

Serious adverse experiences must be reported promptly to the Sponsor. A serious AE is defined as any adverse drug experience occurring at any dose that results in any of the following outcomes: death; a life-threatening adverse drug experience; in-patient hospitalization or prolongation of existing hospitalization; a persistent or significant disability/incapacity; or a congenital anomaly/birth defect. An important medical event that may not result in death, be life-threatening, or require hospitalization may be considered a serious adverse drug experience when, based upon appropriate medical judgment, the event may jeopardize the patient and may require medical or surgical intervention to prevent one of the outcomes listed in this definition.

An adverse experience can meet the definition of a serious AE and, ultimately, not be related to the study drug. In the event of a serious adverse experience, the Sponsor has 10 working days during which to file a Drug Experience Report via the MedWatch Adverse Experience Form (see Appendix II, Form 4) to the FDA. The MedWatch form is part of an overall program designed to streamline the reporting of AEs and product defects associated with medications, devices, and nutritional products. These reports are essential to FDA drug surveillance efforts. MedWatch forms can be obtained from the Sponsor or directly from the FDA (1-800-FDA-1088). To complete the MedWatch form, the Sponsor will need the following information from the CRC:

- ✔ subject's initials, study number, age, and sex;

- ✔ adverse experience reported, all relevant tests and laboratory data, and the status of the reaction to date;

- ✔ dates of test article administration, from the first dose to the time of adverse experience;

- ✔ whether the test article was discontinued and, if so, whether the reaction stopped;

- ✔ whether test article administration was resumed and, if so, whether the reaction reappeared;

- ✔ whether the Investigator believed the experience was related to the test article; and

- ✔ any other factors the investigator considers to be relevant (e.g., concomitant drugs, history, and/or diagnosis).

The PI is also obligated to report in writing serious adverse experiences to the IRB within *10* working days. Some IRBs will require a written report within 24 to 48 hours. Make sure you review the IRB's reporting requirements.

Any abnormal laboratory values, abnormal clinical findings, or adverse experiences that the PI considers to be clinically significant must be medically managed until resolved. Follow-up information should be transmitted regularly to the CRA.

Note: If a patient dies while participating in a clinical trial, a copy of the death certificate may be required. Therefore, it is wise to obtain and have one in the CRC's files.

F. Specimen Handling and Submission Forms

The collection of biologic specimens for shipment to a reference-testing laboratory will be required by most Protocols. Common specimens include plasma, serum, urine, and tissue. The Protocol will provide specific methods for their collection, preservation, and shipping. The Sponsor will supply instructions for the identification and storage of these specimens as well as the necessary submission forms to be completed at the time of shipment.

It is the responsibility of the Investigator and CRC to see that specimens are collected and stored as required by the Protocol. Labels and forms identifying the subject, type of specimens collected, site of collection, and date and time of collection are to be completed at the time of the procedure by the Investigator or designee. Incomplete, missing, or wrong information recorded on a laboratory requisition form may result in a delay in receiving laboratory reports. It is very important to complete the laboratory requisition form according to the instructions provided by the laboratory.

A complete review of specimen collection and handling procedures usually takes place with the Investigator and staff before initiation of the study. In the event that the Sponsor is using a central laboratory, the central laboratory will provide the site's staff with a manual that is study-specific, including instructions for specimen collection and shipment.

G. The Subject Enrollment Form

The Subject Enrollment Form serves many purposes. It provides a checklist of the CRF documents to be completed for each visit and serves as a record of those components of the CRF that have been completed and submitted to the CRO/SMO or CRA. In addition, the Subject Enrollment Form is an aid in scheduling subject visits, as well as providing the status of enrollment activities at each site to the Sponsor.

H. The Site Visit Log (Monitor Log)

The Site Visit Log (Monitor Log) is used to record visits made to the study site by the Sponsor's authorized representative, usually the CRA or a CRO/SMO representative. At each visit, the visitor will sign the Site Visit Log. This log must be kept in the Study File. Should the FDA audit the study, the FDA inspector will want to review the Site Visit Log to determine the frequency of site visits made by the Sponsor and the CRO/SMO, if applicable.

I. The Telephone Log

The Telephone Log is used to record all telephone contacts pertaining to the study. In addition to the date and time, the items discussed, action taken, and follow-up required should also be included.

In some instances, the Sponsor will not require a site visit follow-up letter. In these cases, the CRA may contact the site after the visit to discuss the visit. Record this conversation in the Telephone Log; some CRAs will date and initial this telephone conversation as accurate during their next monitoring visit. As with the Site Visit Log, the Telephone Log should also be kept in the Study File. A sample Telephone Conversation Record is provided in Appendix II (Form 8).

J. Delegation of Authority Log

The Delegation of Authority Log is usually required for the purpose of identifying what study-specific tasks have been delegated by the PI. This is an ICH requirement.

IX. The Prestudy Site Visit

Before investigational products can be sent to the study site and subject enrollment can begin, an initial site visit is conducted by a representative of the Sponsor and the CRO/SMO, if applicable. This is called the prestudy site visit. Sponsors are now utilizing the prestudy visit as a tool to ensure the facility is appropriate for study. In some cases the prestudy visit may be waived according to the Sponsor requirements, e.g., prior studies with the Sponsor with a specific time frame (six months to one year).

A. Site Initiation Visit

The purpose of this visit is to give the Sponsor's representative the opportunity to review the study purpose, intended study patients and some of the study documents, particularly the Investigator Brochure, Protocol, and CRFs, with the PI and staff. The Investigator Brochure is a document that summarizes all clinical and scientific information about the investigational product to date. One of its purposes is to inform investigators of the pharmacologic events and side effects that have been observed in past studies. The Protocol gives specific instructions for the conduct of the study. During the prestudy site visit, the Sponsor's representative will discuss the Protocol and its CRFs page by page. In addition, the Sponsor's representative will outline study procedures, inspect the facilities, and verify safe, secure, and appropriate storage of the investigational product. A representative of the CRO/SMO involved in the study may also be a participant in this review. It is important for the Sponsor or the Sponsor Representative to tour all departments as well as all facilities, including those off site that will be used in the conduct of the clinical trial.

Many studies are using the internet for study contact via emails and will often send documents via internet to the PI.

and CRC. With many studies using electronic CRFs, it is sometimes crucial to the study that the CRC and monitor have access to a high-speed internet connection to enter study data and also to allow routine communications.

At the conclusion of this visit, if everything has met the approval of the Sponsor, you will be invited to participate in the clinical trial. In some cases, the Sponsor representative may ask for copies of the PI and sub- investigator CVs, medical licenses, local lab normals and CLIA, CAP certificates, and IRB meeting dates and study submission requirements. The Sponsor representative may also request a site contact for contract review, budgets and other documents.

X. Recruiting and Enrolling Subjects

The first step in initiating the actual clinical study enrollment is to obtain a list of potential subjects. This can be accomplished by examining subject listings from various sources and by publicizing the study. Examples are given here.

A. Prospective Subject Groups

Lists of prospective subjects can be obtained from the following:

✔ charts in physicians' offices;

✔ computer printouts by diagnosis from hospital clinic records;

✔ support groups;

✔ group screening records;

✔ clinical laboratory screening records;

✔ SMO specializing in the identification of Protocol specific potential subjects; and

✔ referrals from physicians, nurses, coordinators, and other specialty areas (e.g., radiology, laboratory), with a referral fee offered.

B. Methods of Publicizing the Study

A clinical study can be advertised or publicized in a variety of ways. However, IRB and Sponsor approval are required in advance for newspaper, radio, and television advertising and for any signs that are to be posted in public places, such as waiting rooms (see Appendix II, Form 9 for a sample sign). The following are several methods by which patients may learn about the availability of a clinical study:

✔ advertising (newspaper, radio, television);

✔ signs/posters for waiting areas;

✔ quarterly newsletter to subjects;

✔ billing statements;

✔ Kiwanis, Lions Clubs, Rotary Clubs, or other community groups;

- ✔ local churches and daycare centers;

- ✔ subject information in waiting rooms/examination areas;

- ✔ health fairs;

- ✔ local colleges and universities; and

- ✔ notices to local support groups for specific diseases.

Several states, including Florida, have enacted laws for advertisements by healthcare providers of free or discounted services. These laws require that specific language be included in study-related advertisements. To see if your state has enacted a law similar to the one enacted by the state of Florida, contact the appropriate agency in your state from which you may obtain this information. The following is the Florida Statute:

Florida Statutes Chapter 455.664

Advertisement by a Health Care Provider of Free or Discounted Services; Required Statement

In any advertisement for a free, discounted fee, or reduced fee service, examination, or treatment by a health care provider licensed under chapter 458, chapter 459, chapter 460, chapter 461, chapter 462, chapter 463, chapter 464, chapter 466, or chapter 486, the following statement shall appear in capital letters clearly distinguishable from the rest of the text:

THE PATIENT AND ANY OTHER PERSON RESPONSIBLE FOR PAYMENT HAS A RIGHT TO REFUSE TO PAY, CANCEL PAYMENT, OR BE REIMBURSED FOR PAYMENT FOR ANY OTHER SERVICE, EXAMINATION, OR TREATMENT THAT IS PERFORMED AS A RESULT OF AND WITHIN 72 HOURS OF RESPONDING TO THE ADVERTISEMENT FOR THE FREE, DISCOUNTED FEE, OR REDUCED FEE SERVICE, EXAMINATION, OR TREATMENT.

However, the required statement shall not be necessary as an accompaniment to an advertisement of a licensed health care provider defined by this section if the advertisement appears in a classified directory, the primary purpose of which is to provide products and services at free, reduced, or discounted prices to consumers and in which the statement prominently appears in at least one place.

Added by Laws 1997, c.97-261,x 81, eff. July 1, 1997

However, if the advertisement does not state "free" or "at no cost," the statement is not required. Check with your IRB for further clarification.

C. Presenting the Study to the Subject

Once a list of potential subjects has been obtained, the CRC must screen the subjects for acceptability and introduce them to the details of the study. This can be accomplished by telephone or in person.

When first contacting or meeting a potential study subject, the CRC should give his/her name and affiliation with the clinic or physician conducting the study. The reasons for conducting the current study should be explained, and an investigational drug study should be defined, if appropriate. That is, the subject should understand that the drug has been previously used in humans, but additional human data are needed before the drug may be introduced to the marketplace.

The subject is then screened according to the inclusion/exclusion criteria set forth in the study Protocol. If the subject meets the criteria, the CRC can outline the details of the study more fully.

The potential benefits and possible side effects of the study drug should be discussed. The subject should be made fully aware of the time commitment required, the need to administer the test article as instructed, the need to follow the Protocol, and the importance of compliance. The length of the study, the number of on-site visits needed, and the procedures that will be performed at each visit should be fully outlined.

If the subject has been contacted by telephone, an appointment should be made for him/her to come in to review and sign the informed consent form. If the subject has been contacted in person, informed consent can be obtained at this visit. The subject must review the informed consent form and then be encouraged to ask any questions regarding the study and informed consent. The subject then signs the form with the CRC acting as witness. (A duly authorized representative may act on behalf of the subject.) The PI's signature will also be obtained on this form.

Once informed consent has been obtained, the subject's next appointment (typically the baseline screening visit) should be scheduled. The subject should be given the CRC's name and phone number. The subject also receives a copy of the informed consent form, any study overview, and a confirmation letter (see Appendix II, Form 11), if appropriate.

It is the responsibility of the CRC and Investigator to ensure that a clinical study has been completed with the designated number of clinically acceptable subjects and that these subjects report for every scheduled visit. Therefore, when first presenting a study to a potential subject, it is important to point out the benefits of study participation. These might include the following key points:

- ✔ preferential treatment, including convenient appointment times, no delays getting in for a scheduled appointment, ample appointment time, confirmation calls for next visit, follow-up calls and letters, transportation provided if needed, personalized appraisal of laboratory test results, and thorough healthcare;

- ✔ free medical and laboratory tests (e.g., electrocardiogram, chest radiographs, and blood and urine analyses);

- ✔ possible monetary compensation for travel expenses;

- ✔ opportunity to participate in innovative drug research;

- ✔ opportunity to possibly help others; and

- ✔ opportunity to increase understanding about disease processes.

To ensure fair balance, the subject must also be made aware of the potential risks involved in participating in the study.

On occasion, a subject will require special instructions about a particular procedure or test. The following box provides an example of one such special information directive.

Instructions for 24-Hour Urine Collection

The same amount of liquids should be consumed during the collection period as are normally consumed. No alcoholic or caffeine-containing beverages (coffee, tea, cola) may be consumed during this period.

The collection starts *after* you empty your bladder in the morning. *(The urine voided at this time is not included in the collection.)* Write the time and date on the label of the specimen container. Collect all urine voided for the next 24 hours in this one container, including the first specimen voided the following morning.

The specimen container should be refrigerated during the collection period. Each voiding should be added to the container as soon as possible.

Proper collection and refrigeration of the urine specimen is very important for accurate test results. Please follow the above directions and call me if you have any questions.

[Name]
Clinical Research Coordinator

[Phone number]

XI. Conducting the Study and Keeping Records

A. Study Activities

All the work performed up to this point should facilitate the accurate and timely transfer of study data to the CRFs. However, while the clinical study is being conducted, the CRC must ensure that clinical findings and laboratory data are properly recorded. Toward this end, the CRC should:

- ✔ organize and label specimen containers;
- ✔ prepare all laboratory requisition sheets;
- ✔ prepare Subject Workfolders before each visit;
- ✔ oversee the receipt and handling of test articles and laboratory specimens;
- ✔ maintain all files, records, and logs;
- ✔ prepare for site visits; and
- ✔ schedule appointments during the monitoring visits for the pharmacy and/or laboratory if required.

For a study to be successful, *the Protocol must be followed and subject numbers maintained.* Some common pitfalls to avoid follow.

Lack of Timely Treatment. This may occur, leading to subject withdrawal if the physician's office

staff is not alerted to the status of a study subject. To avoid this problem, the names of study participants should be highlighted in the physician's appointment book.

Laboratory Specimens Not Analyzed. Laboratory specimens must be processed within a certain period of time to meet the requirements of the laboratory or the Protocol. If specimens are not processed in a timely manner, the Protocol may be violated or important laboratory data may have to be excluded. When possible, a back-up sample should be retained.

Subject Absence. Subjects must show up for the required number of office visits, as dictated by the Protocol. To minimize subject absence, the CRC should telephone or mail a post-card to remind the subject of the upcoming appointment.

B. Subjects Lost to Follow-Up

If a subject is continually absent for appointments, the CRC should try to contact him/her by phone or certified letter to determine any scheduling conflicts and, if possible, reschedule the missed appointments. If attempts at follow-up using the informed consent form and/or letters of agreement fail to convince the subject to report for scheduled appointments, the subject must be withdrawn from the study. If this is the case, every attempt should be made to have the test articles returned to the study site. The dates the subject was contacted and the type of contact used should be recorded in the study documentation.

C. Withdrawing a Subject

A subject may be withdrawn (terminated) from a study for several reasons, including failure to follow the Protocol or having an adverse reaction to the test article. A subject may also voluntarily withdraw. In the event a subject is withdrawn, a final visit should be scheduled, and the Sponsor should be notified of the subject's withdrawal. The subject's randomization code should not be broken at this time except in the case of an emergency. Many study Protocols require follow-up to be continued for a specified period of time after a subject is withdrawn, regardless of the reason for withdrawal.

D. Site Visits During the Study

The study site will be visited several times by the CRA or representative of the CRO/SMO. The complexity of the study or the number of subjects enrolled will dictate the number of visits. In addition, the CRA will monitor the study site by telephone. At each telephone contact or site visit, the CRA will confer with the CRC and the PI regarding the progress of the study.

During a typical site visit, the CRA is required to perform the tasks that follow. A review of these items will help the CRC prepare for the CRA's site visit.

Sign Site Visit Log (Monitoring Log). All of the Sponsor's personnel must sign the log each day they visit the study site.

Inspect original, signed informed consent forms. These must be available for all subjects enrolled since the CRA's previous site visit.

Inspect CRFs. CRFs must be completed legibly using a black ballpoint pen or typewriter. They must be available for review within two weeks after the subject completes the study.

Inspect Applicable Source Documents. The CRA will check for:

> ✔ properly completed entries;

✔ consistency between CRFs (all laboratory data and at least 20 percent of all other entries will be checked against source documents; most studies involve a 100 percent quality control check);

✔ conformity with the Protocol; and

✔ properly signed and dated CRFs (these must be signed by the PI or the authorized designee).

Inspect Test Article Storage Area. The CRA will require access to this area to ensure that:

✔ adequate supplies are on hand;

✔ test articles are being stored properly;

✔ the Drug Accountability Record is being properly maintained;

✔ there is agreement amongst a physical count of the test articles received versus the number of test articles dispensed (as recorded on the Drug Accountability Record and CRFs) versus the number of test articles on hand;

✔ there is agreement between the dispensing record and the CRFs regarding the identification of subjects receiving the test article; and

✔ all test articles returned by subjects have been accurately counted and recorded on the Drug Accountability Record.

Inspect Bioanalytical and Specimen Storage Area. The CRA will need access to this area to ensure that samples collected since the last visit have been properly collected, handled, and stored.

E. Closing the Study and Retaining Records

At the termination of the study or at the request of the Sponsor, the CRA or representative of the CRO/SMO will pick up all remaining supplies and the final Drug Accountability Record for transmittal to the Sponsor. A copy of the Drug Accountability Record will be retained in the Study File.

Study Close-Out Checklist. At the close of a study, the CRC is required to:

✔ schedule a close-out meeting with the Sponsor;

✔ notify the IRB of close-out and submit a final report;

✔ submit a final report to the Sponsor;

✔ submit miscellaneous charges to the Sponsor;

✔ return or discard laboratory supplies;

✔ bind and store CRFs;

✔ return or discard unused CRFs;

✔ label and ship frozen specimens;

✔ complete and store audit file;

✔ request randomization information; and

✔ track disbursements and reconcile study finances with the Sponsor.

IRB Final Report. The IRB Final Report is submitted after all the subjects have completed the study. This is sent to the IRB, with a copy sent to the Sponsor.

Record Retention. Federal law requires that the PI retain all study records for two years following the NDA approval date. The Sponsor may request longer retention periods. If the application is not approved, or no NDA is submitted, the PI must retain all study records for at least two years after the FDA has been notified that all clinical investigations of this indication have been discontinued. The ICH guidelines recommend that the records be retained for 15 years. When archiving study records, clearly label the following:

✔ Protocol number;

✔ Sponsor name;

✔ Investigator name;

✔ Investigator address; and

✔ study close-out date.

The PI must obtain the written consent of the Sponsor before disposing of any study records.

Subject Follow-Up. Subjects appreciate receiving correspondence after a study has been completed. You may wish to send them a letter describing the drug group in which they participated, provide a self-assessment form so they may rate their satisfaction with the conduct of the study, or thank them for their participation.

XII. Preparing for an FDA Audit

A. FDA Inspections of Clinical Trials

The FDA Bioresearch Monitoring Program involves site visits to PIs, research Sponsors, CROs/SMOs, IRBs, and nonclinical (animal) laboratories. All FDA product areas such as drugs, biologics, medical devices, radiological products, foods, and veterinary drugs are involved in the Bioresearch Monitoring Program. The program procedures are dependent upon the product type. The objective of all FDA inspections is to ensure the integrity and quality of data and information submitted to the FDA, as well as the protection of human research subjects.

The FDA carries out three distinct types of clinical trial inspections:

- ✔ study-oriented inspections;
- ✔ PI-oriented inspections; and
- ✔ bioequivalence study inspections.

Study-Oriented Inspections

FDA field offices conduct study-oriented inspections based on assignments developed by headquarters staff. Assignments are based almost exclusively on studies that are important to product evaluation, such as NDAs and product license applications pending before the FDA.

When a PI who has participated in the study being examined is selected for an inspection, the FDA investigator from the FDA district office will contact the PI to schedule a mutually acceptable time for the inspection.

Upon arrival at the site, the FDA investigator will show FDA credentials, consisting of a photo identification, and present a Notice of Inspection Form to the PI. FDA credentials let the PI know that the investigator is a duly authorized representative of the FDA.

If, during the course of an FDA inspection, a PI has any questions that the FDA investigator has not answered, either the director of the district office or the center that initiated the inspection may be contacted. The name and telephone number of the district director and the specific center contact person are available from the FDA investigator.

B. Types of FDA Inspections

There are two main types of FDA inspections that you are likely to encounter: a routine inspection and a for-cause inspection.

A *routine* inspection is conducted for those studies that are crucial to a product's evaluation and approval. For example, the studies may be pivotal to an NDA pending before the FDA. As the name would imply, a *for-cause* inspection is conducted when the FDA has a specific reason (cause) for inspecting a study site. The reason might be one of the following: (1) an Investigator has participated in a large number of studies; (2) an Investigator has done work outside his/her specialty; (3) the safety or efficacy results of an Investigator are inconsistent with those of others conducting the same study; or (4) the Investigator claims too many subjects with a specific disease or indication compared with the low numbers associated with his/her practice. Numerous other reasons determined by the FDA may trigger a for-cause inspection.

Before an inspection, the FDA will contact the PI, usually through a letter, to schedule the date of inspection and to determine the specific material to be audited. After receiving notice of a pending inspection, the PI should immediately contact the CRA because the Sponsor may wish to meet with site personnel prior to the FDA inspection.

The FDA inspector will present FDA credentials and a completed Form FDA 482, Notice of Inspection. (This form can be located on the FDA website.) The CRC should reserve a private area for the inspector, such as a conference room, and organize all appropriate source documents for the inspection. The inspector should have access to all, and only, the study data that was specifically requested, nothing more and nothing less. In addition, the following related information should be available:

- ✔ physicians' office records;
- ✔ hospital records;
- ✔ laboratory test results;
- ✔ subject medical history;
- ✔ subject follow-up data; and
- ✔ appointment calendar.

The inspector may also request the following information:

- ✔ the degree of delegation of authority by the PI;
- ✔ how and where data were recorded;
- ✔ how test article accountability was administered and maintained;

- ✔ how the Sponsor communicated with the PI and evaluated the study program; and

- ✔ certification of service/calibration for study-related equipment.

C. Parts of the Investigation

The investigation consists of two basic parts. The first is determining the facts surrounding the conduct of the study, including:

- ✔ who did what during the conduct of the clinical trial;

- ✔ the degree of delegation of authority performed by the PI— whether they were properly supervised and had the experience to do the assigned task;

- ✔ where specific aspects of the study were performed;

- ✔ if they are listed in the FDA 1572;

- ✔ how and where the data were recorded;

- ✔ how test article accountability was dispensed and maintained;

- ✔ how the CRA communicated with the clinical investigator; and

- ✔ how the CRA monitor evaluated the progress of the clinical trial.

Second, the clinical trial data is audited. The FDA investigator compares the data submitted to the FDA and/or the Sponsor with all available records that might support the data. These records may come from the physician's office, hospital, nursing home, central and/or local laboratories, and other sources. The FDA may also examine patient records that predate the study to determine whether the medical condition being studied was, in fact, properly diagnosed and whether an interfering medication had possibly been given before the study began. The FDA investigator may also review records covering a reasonable period after completion of the clinical trial to determine if there was proper follow-up, and if all signs and symptoms reasonably attributable to the product's use had been reported.

Principal Investigator-Oriented Inspections

A PI-oriented inspection may be initiated because a PI conducted a pivotal study that merits in-depth examination because of its singular importance in product approval or its effect on medical practice. An inspection may also be initiated because representatives of the Sponsor have reported to the FDA that they are having some difficulty getting case reports from the PI, or that the FDA has some other concern with the PI's work.

In addition, the FDA may initiate an inspection if a subject in a study complains about the Protocol or human subject's rights violations.

PI-oriented inspections may also be initiated because:

- ✔ the PI participated in a large number of studies;
- ✔ the PI enrolled a significantly large number of subjects into a Protocol;
- ✔ the PI participated in clinical trials outside of his/her specialty areas;
- ✔ the safety or effectiveness findings were inconsistent with those of other PIs studying the same test article;
- ✔ too many subjects with a specific disease given the locale of the investigations were claimed; and/or
- ✔ the laboratory results were outside the range of expected biological variation.

Once the FDA determines that a PI-oriented inspection should be conducted, the procedures are essentially the same as in the study-oriented inspection, except that the data audit goes into greater depth, covers more case reports, and may cover more than one study. If the Investigator has repeatedly or deliberately violated FDA regulations or has submitted false information to the Sponsor in a required report, the FDA will initiate actions that may ultimately decide that the PI is not to receive investigational products in the future.

Bioequivalence Study Inspections

A bioequivalence study inspection differs from the other inspections in that it requires participation by an FDA chemist or a PI who is knowledgeable about analytical evaluations.

D. Preparation and Instructions for an FDA Audit

The PI is responsible for *all* aspects of the clinical trial. When the PI signs the FDA Form 1572, he/she is making a commitment to the FDA. One of those commitments is to permit regulatory inspections.

When arranging a routine audit of a site, the FDA will generally contact the site by telephone two to three weeks in advance to schedule a time and date that is convenient.

In a for-cause audit conducted by the FDA (including audits of Sponsors or CROs), the FDA generally will show up unannounced. If this should ever occur at your site, remember you cannot legally prohibit the FDA from conducting its audit. In addition, it will be necessary to contact every Sponsor with whom you are conducting a Protocol to inform them of the for-cause audit.

Prior to the FDA Audit

The PI and his/her staff generally meet to discuss the audit and to organize the information and records requested by the FDA inspectors.

The following items should be available *before* the FDA inspectors arrive:

- ✔ Original, signed informed consent forms for all subjects, including those randomized as well as screen failures, including all signed versions of the informed consent

- ✔ Completed CRFs for all subjects randomized, as well as screen failures

- ✔ Source documents and any other subject charts, including medical charts, laboratory reports, radiology reports, EKGs, etc.

- ✔ All versions of the Investigator Brochure

- ✔ All versions of the Protocol and Protocol Amendments

- ✔ All study drug receipt records, dispensing records, and return records

- ✔ Complete and current Regulatory Binder

The FDA Audit

Upon arrival of the FDA inspector, request identification and obtain a business card or record his/her name, title, division office, and contact number. The FDA inspector will present a Form FDA 482 (Notice of Intent to Audit), which presents the clinical trial to be audited and the scope of the audit. It is important to identify a room or office for the FDA inspector to work in while conducting the audit.

Pointers

The following pointers may be helpful to remember during the FDA audit:

- ✔ Use the same room throughout the audit.

- ✔ Ensure the room has a telephone.

- ✔ Provide *only requested* clinical trial records.

- ✔ Ensure there are no records for any other clinical trial in the room designated as the room for the FDA inspector.

- ✔ If there are any cabinets, drawers, or cupboard in the room, ensure they are locked.

- ✔ Periodically check with the FDA inspector during the audit, instead of remaining in the room during the audit.

- ✔ Designate a contact person who can address questions, provide administrative support, track all requests from the auditor, and make photocopies, if appropriate.

- ✔ Document the records requested by the FDA auditor, the questions asked and the answers provided, as well as the name of the person providing the answers.

✔ Ensure the FDA auditor is escorted by site personnel at *all times* during the audit.

✔ Remember, the policy for FDA inspections, as well as Sponsor audits, is set by the PI or the written SOPs in place at your site.

✔ Notify the medical records department and pharmacy if applicable and any other administrative offices.

✔ Notify the IRB prior to the audit.

Be prepared to discuss the following items in detail:

✔ The informed consent process, including the person(s) responsible for obtaining written informed consent from the subject.

✔ The process for recruiting patients for the clinical trial.

✔ Delegation of responsibilities by the PI.

✔ The CRF completion process.

✔ SAEs reporting process and the reporting requirements for the IRB.

✔ How the PI maintains his/her oversight of the clinical trial.

✔ Concurrent clinical trials.

✔ Subjects who have discontinued the clinical trial being audited and subsequently may have been enrolled into another clinical trial.

✔ If an extension study is being audited, be prepared to provide the informed consent for the parent clinical trial for all subjects who have entered the extension study (the FDA auditor may only be verifying the subject signatures).

✔ Frequency of monitoring visits and how long the monitor stayed at the site during each visit.

✔ Study drug randomization and kit/bottle assignments.

✔ If an automated drug randomization process was used, ensure all related documents are available (including fax confirmations).

✔ Study drug accountability including overall and individual subject records.

✔ Ensure the area where the study drug is being stored is secure (locked) and there is limited access to the area.

✔ Ensure study drug not dispensed is being kept separate from study drug that has been returned/dispensed.

✔ Document any study drug discrepancies, including study drug containers inadvertently discarded by the patient.

✔ Ensure there is written documentation for the process of transporting study drug from one center to another, if applicable.

When the audit has been completed, the FDA auditor may issue the following documents:

✔ Form FDA 483 (Inspectional Observations) used for violations of the Federal Regulations. A Form FDA 483 is not always issued when the FDA conducts an audit; however, it is difficult *not* to get one.

✔ Establishment Inspection Report (EIR).

The Exit Interview

Appoint one person to provide comprehensive documentation of the information from the FDA auditor's exit interview with the PI. The person designated should not be distracted by participating in the discussion. Remember tape recorders and video tape recorders are not permitted. The following information should be documented:

✔ Document each observation provided in the Form FDA 483.

✔ Make sure the observation is understood.

✔ Point out any deficiency noted in the observation that has been corrected since the beginning of the FDA audit (perhaps the observation will be deleted from the Form FDA 483, but that is not always likely).

✔ If the corrected observation has not been deleted from the Form FDA 483, request that the FDA auditor's Form FDA 483 and EIR include the fact that the observation noted has been corrected.

✔ If any observation noted deals with not meeting FDA regulations, *carefully* point out that the regulations are subject to interpretation, and, if correct, that "our interpretation was intended to provide the greatest protection to our patients."

✔ If it is clear that corrective action is necessary on an observation, and it is clear what the action to be taken is, indicate that you plan to take appropriate corrective measures on that observation immediately.

✔ *Do not commit yourself* to a future action that you do not intend to make or cannot undertake.

✔ If the corrective action is underway, but not completed with respect to a noted observation, report that fact to the FDA auditor.

✔ If you believe a noted observation is clearly not warranted, you should also point that out in a diplomatic manner.

✔ Set the proper tone.

✔ Be aware of your rights and protect them.

✔ Being argumentative will not be constructive and could make things worse.

✔ The primary focus is to clearly understand the observation(s) and address the observation(s).

✔ Do not be upset or offended if you do receive a Form FDA 483.

✔ If you respond within 10 working days of receipt of the Form FDA 483, your response will become part of the original report that is provided upon request of that report through the Freedom of Information Services.

✔ Remember, Form FDA 483 and EIRs are requested by Sponsors and CROs routinely.

General Advice

A few tips to make the process less painful:

✔ The more cooperative and the better prepared you are, the faster and more smoothly the inspection will proceed.

✔ Only answer the questions asked—*do not volunteer* any additional information.

✔ Do not be afraid to say "I don't know, but I will find out and get back to you," then do so—promptly.

✔ If you are not sure how to answer a question, say "I will have to get back to you on that," then obtain the appropriate advice on how to answer the question.

✔ If you don't feel comfortable answering a question, say "I will have to get back to you on that," then obtain appropriate advice on how to answer the question.

✔ Do not refuse to answer any question or provide anything; if you are not comfortable or cannot or do not want to answer the question, say, "I'll have to check with Dr. Z regarding that request."

✔ Try not to be overly friendly—remember what they are there to do; they may interpret your actions differently than you intended them.

✔ Know what you are talking about *before* you say anything and make sure you can back it up with documentation.

✔ You are free to call the Sponsor or CRO with any questions or concerns at any time during the inspection process (it is important to stay in close contact with the Sponsor/CRO).

✔ Remember, at the close-out visit for each of your studies, make sure you keep the project contact information. Clients should provide the names and telephone numbers of contacts to be called after the site receives the initial call from the FDA or other Regulatory Authority.

✔ Regulatory Authority inspections occur most frequently from six months up to two years following an NDA, BLA, or MAA (Marketing Approval Application) submission.

Summary

It is important to have written policies and SOPs in place for handling any FDA and client/CRO audits/inspections:

✔ Make sure all staff members know how to handle such audits and that they have been trained in the SOPs.

✔ Make sure training records for your staff members are current and accurate.

✔ Be courteous at all times.

✔ When or if it is appropriate, request a teleconference with the inspector/auditor's supervisor.

✔ Be sure you understand all observations and findings.

✔ Answer all questions briefly, concisely, and truthfully (don't ever think the auditor/inspector will not find out the real answer).

✔ Visit FDA websites to read warning letters for Sponsors, PIs, and Ethics Committees (there are several website addresses in this handbook).

E. Common FDA Inspection Findings

At the end of an investigation, the FDA investigator will conduct an "exit interview" with the clinical investigator. During this interview, the FDA investigator will discuss the findings from the inspection with the PI. The FDA investigator will clarify any misunderstandings that might exist and may issue a written Form FDA 483 (Notice of Observations) to the PI. Following the inspection, the FDA field investigator will prepare a written report and submit it to headquarters for evaluation.

Once the report has been evaluated, the FDA headquarters usually issues a letter to the PI. The letter is generally one of three types:

Notice that no significant deviations from the regulations were observed. This letter does not require any response from the PI.

Informational letter that identifies deviations from the Code of Federal Regulations and GCP. This letter may or may not require a response from the PI. If a response is requested, the letter will describe what is necessary and provide a contact person for clarification or further questions.

Warning letter that identifies deviations from the Code of Federal Regulations requiring prompt correction by the PI. This letter will provide the PI with a contact person for clarification and questions. In these cases, the FDA may inform both the Sponsor and the reviewing IRB of the deficiencies. The FDA may also inform the Sponsor if the PI's procedural deficiencies indicate ineffective monitoring by the Sponsor. In addition to issuing these warning letters, the FDA may take other courses of action, which may include regulatory, legal, and/or administrative sanctions.

Office for Human Research Protections

In June 2000, the FDA announced the creation of a new office at the Department of Health and Human Services (HHS), the Office for Human Research Protections (OHRP), to lead efforts for protecting human subjects in biomedical and behavioral research. This office replaces the Office for Protection from Research Risks (OPRR), which was part of the National Institute of Health. The OPRR had authority over NIH-funded research.

According to the HHS Assistant Secretary, this new office will have increased resources and broader responsibility to ensure that patients taking part in research are better protected and fully informed. Everyone in the research community must share the responsibility for protecting research subjects. Medical research today is exploding with opportunity; however, to achieve the benefits of that research, we need a solid foundation of thoughtfully designed and thoroughly executed research-patient protection. This new OHRP will work with HHS agencies, research institutions, and Sponsors of research to ensure that this foundation is in place and working productively.

For additional information, a copy of the FDA *Compliance Program Guidance Manual* for Clinical Investigator Inspections (Program 7348.811), the document issued by the FDA investigator to conduct the inspection, is available by writing to:

Freedom of Information Staff (HFI-30)
Federal Food and Drug Administration
5600 Fishers Lane
Rockville, MD 20857

In addition, see the FDA information sheet, "Clinical Investigator Regulatory Sanctions," available at the FDA website.

F. Common Problems Identified in Audits of Clinical Trials

Audit Problem Areas	Items for Caution
Protocol	Under what Protocol date did the site initiate the study? If there are several versions, is the initiation version at the site and is it documented that this is the appropriate Protocol version? In addition, are all versions of the Protocol in the Investigator File?
Protocol Signature Page	Are corresponding completed signature pages provided for all versions of the Protocol?
Investigator Brochure (IB)	What version of the IB was provided to the site? Was the IB revised during the clinical trial? Is there documentation showing that the IB was received by the site (e.g., a memo to the Investigator File stating when the document was sent or a monitoring report listing the document as being at the site)? Where is the IB kept? If it is not kept in the Investigator File, is there a memo stating where at the site the IB can be located?
Form FDA 1572	Has the form been correctly completed, signed, and dated? If there is more than one form with the same signature/date, which form is correct? Has section #8 been appropriately completed? If Form FDA 1572 has been revised, was a copy sent to the IRB as well as the Sponsor?
Curriculum Vitae (CV)	Does the site have a CV for each person listed on FDA Form 1572? Does the site have a current medical license for the PI (some Sponsors require a copy of the medical license for the subinvestigator(s) as well as the PI)? Are all CVs current within two years? Can this be easily determined by review of the CV? Does the CV document the PI's affiliation with the site conducting the clinical trial?
Confidentiality Agreement	Was the Confidentiality Agreement obtained prior to the release of all study-related documentation (e.g., protocol, IB, Financial Disclosure form)?
Informed Consent Forms	Is there a copy of the IRB approved consent on file? Does the IRB documentation indicate that it is approving the consent? Has the informed consent been revised? Was the revised consent forwarded to the IRB? Is there documentation indicating that revised consent was approved? Have the patients participating in the Protocol signed the correct version of the informed consent? Are all sections of the informed consent signed and dated appropriately? If the site has foreign-speaking patients, is there a copy of the translated IRB approved consent? Has a certified translator completed the translation? Is there a back translation showing exactly what information is being presented to the patient? If the study has enrolled minors, is guardian consent obtained? If appropriate, is there assent by the minor participating in the Protocol? If there is another individual signing for the patient (e.g., daughter signs for father or wife signs for husband), is the individual the legal representative of the subject? If this is an in-hospital clinical trial, has the hospital's requirements for a legal representative been met? Has the reason there is another individual signing the informed consent for the patient been documented? Have all informed consent documents been signed prior to the initiation of any study-related screening procedures (e.g., medication wash-out periods, fasting for screening laboratory tests)?
Serious Adverse Events	Have all serious adverse events been reported to the Sponsor, CRO/SMO, and IRB within the specified time frames? Does the documentation provide a complete picture of the event? Has the condition been followed until resolution? In the event the patient has died, is there a copy of the death certificate in the source documents?
Institutional Review Board (IRB)	Does the site have documentation that the IRB is appropriately formed (e.g., membership list or assurance number)? Can all IRB approvals be easily tracked to the corresponding study document? Are there periodic reviews being appropriately submitted to the IRB and in a timely fashion? Is there documentation in the Investigator File from the IRB in response to the reviews? Are study summaries sent to the IRB upon study completion? Are all serious adverse events being appropriately reported? Are significant Protocol departures being reported to the IRB? Is there documentation in the Investigator File from the IRB in response to the reports?

Audit Problem Areas	Items for Caution
Site Visit Follow-Up Documentation	Are issues identified during a site-monitoring visit followed up in subsequent visits? Is there documentation to indicate that identified issues have been appropriately resolved?
Laboratory Documentation	Does the site have the appropriate laboratory certification (e.g., CLIA, CAP, and state license where applicable)? Does the certification cover the duration of the study? Are there normal laboratory value ranges available? If a central laboratory is being used for the study and there were Protocol samples sent to a local laboratory, is the appropriate certification for both the central and the local laboratories available in the Investigator File?
Investigational Supplies	Can all investigational supplies be accounted for? Are all study-related supplies being appropriately stored (e.g., if test articles need refrigeration, are they stored in a refrigerator with a temperature monitor and log? Is the temperature log current? If the test article is a controlled substance, have the appropriate guidelines for storage and dispensing been performed?)
Site Equipment Specific to the Protocol	Has the equipment being used been serviced recently? Are the service logs available? If calibration is required, has the calibration been performed prior to the initiation of any study-related procedures? Is there documentation of the calibration?
Correspondence	Is there sufficient correspondence between the site and the Sponsor, the site and the IRB, and the site and CRO and/or SMO to demonstrate ongoing communication for the duration of the study? Have all required documentation been forwarded to the IRB, including periodic reports, annual reviews, and study summaries?
Research Charts (Source Documents)	Does the subject's research chart capture sufficient information to demonstrate participation in the clinical trial? Does the information transcribed on the CRFs substantiate the research chart? Are adverse events and serious adverse events recorded in the subject's research chart?

XIII. Clinical Research: Potential Liability

A. Fraud

In clinical research, as in other disciplines, fraud is the deliberate reporting of false or misleading data and/or the withholding of material data, with the intent to mislead the Sponsor, FDA, or any other party that would have an interest in the data. Once the Sponsor has discovered the fraud, the Sponsor should report the PI's misconduct to the IRB and the FDA for further investigation.

Over the past several years, CRCs have also been criminally cited for fraud. One CRC indicated phone calls to subjects specified in the Protocol were noted as having been completed; however, upon review, it was determined the calls noted were never made. The CRC was indicted by the Federal Government, fined, and banned from working on clinical trials.

Types of Fraud

The definition of fraud includes:

✔ the misrepresentation made by the PI and/or his/her representative by words or through conduct;

✔ the misrepresentation made by the PI and/or his/her representative with the knowledge that the representation was not true;

✔ representation made with an intention that should cause the Sponsor to act on it; and

✔ the Sponsor's use of the clinical data collected by this PI and/or his/her representative and damage suffered by use of this data.

Who Can Commit Fraud?

Anyone associated with the collection, transcribing, reporting, or monitoring of clinical trial data can commit fraud. This includes the:

✔ PI;

✔ subinvestigator(s);

✔ Study Coordinator;

✔ CRA;

✔ data manager; and

✔ study patient.

Methods Used by the Pharmaceutical Industry to Detect Fraud

These include:

- ✔ identifying the original source data;
- ✔ verifying the existence and accuracy of the source data;
- ✔ challenging the integrity of the data;
- ✔ tracking missing patient records;
- ✔ recognizing fabricated data that will point in the direction of inconclusive results favoring the test article;
- ✔ observing if all the documents are prepared or written by the same person;
- ✔ noting a repeated pattern of data and identifying departures from anticipated trends;
- ✔ determining if the PI and his/her staff have the expertise, capability, and equipment to perform the clinical trial;
- ✔ determining the sequence of events and considering whether it was physically possible for the individual(s) to perform the work in the given time frame;
- ✔ observing patient diary cards that are overly pristine;
- ✔ noticing that the handwriting is the same or very similar on the diary cards;
- ✔ observing that the same writing implements were used to complete patient diary cards;
- ✔ observing that the data collected during the course of the clinical trial are too perfect;
- ✔ comparing laboratory data for all subjects enrolled in the clinical trial;
- ✔ observing when patients were seen at the site (e.g., if patients were seen on holidays or weekends when it was not required by the design of the clinical trial);
- ✔ noting a lack of AEs, especially in certain patient populations with specific disease indications;
- ✔ noting similar blood pressure results for all patients enrolled in the clinical trial; and
- ✔ comparing returned study medication to determine if there is a pattern to the way the blister packs were opened.

Investigator Misconduct

PI misconduct can be defined as follows:

✔ a flagrant, but nondeliberate violation of the Code of Federal Regulations and GCP guidelines;

✔ modification of the research data to improve
   ✔ ability to publish;
   ✔ accountability;

✔ intentional violation of the code of federal regulations; and

✔ deliberate fabrication of clinical trial results.

B. Negligence

PI negligence can exist when some of the clinical research data are compromised. The compromised data collected by this PI must be removed from the study database and must not be included in the statistical analysis of the clinical trial.

PI negligence can result from:

✔ disorganized data and source documentation;

✔ sloppy record keeping, including source documents; and/or

✔ no or missing documentation.

However, the CRC and the CRA can correct these issues via proper documentation.

PI negligence can exist when the PI has failed to exercise control over the clinical trial in question. In this instance, all the data generated by this PI is compromised and *all* of the efficacy data collected during the conduct of the clinical trial must be removed from the study database and must not be included in the statistical analysis of the clinical trial.

According to an article in the *New York Times* in May 1999, in an era of managed care, the number of private physicians in research since 1990 has almost tripled, and top-enrolling physicians can earn as much as $500,000 to $1 million a year. Pharmaceutical companies and their contractors (CROs/SMOs) offer large payments to physicians and other allied health professionals to encourage them to enroll patients quickly. There are finder's fees paid to physicians for referring their patients to other physicians conducting clinical trials. In some instances, there are payments to everyone involved in the clinical trial who can assist in the recruitment of patients.

Physicians with substantial compensation at stake may persuade patients to take drugs that are inappropriate or even unsafe for them due to pre-existing medical conditions. Unfortunately, clinical research fraud has become a problem in recent years, resulting in the criminal prosecution of several physicians and study coordinators.

Study patients may also commit fraud by providing false information to participate in a specific study. If patient fraud is detected, notify the Sponsor immediately.

C. Legal Liability and the Clinical Research Coordinator

Criminal liability is the violation of statutes that carry criminal penalties. These can be state or federal statutes. The Federal FDA regulates clinical research, and a violation of the regulations could result in federal and state criminal prosecution.

Actions that could result in criminal liability include:

- ✔ intentionally creating false or misleading data for submission to the FDA; and

- ✔ assisting with/covering up intentionally false or misleading data created by a PI for the FDA. It was noted in the *Journal of Good Clinical Practices* that a Study Coordinator was charged for documenting that study-specific telephone calls were made, when in fact the calls were never made. The Study Coordinator was sanctioned, fined, and no longer able to work on clinical trials.

In some instances, a criminal prosecutor may go after a CRC to get the CRC to testify against the PI. *A good rule to follow: If a CRC is asked to do something by the PI and thinks it is or may be wrong, the CRC should not do it!*

Civil liability occurs when deliberate actions, such as fraud, and nondelinquent actions, such as negligence, could result in liability for monetary damages.

A CRC could be considered the agent of the PI if the coordinator performs tasks delegated by the PI. A CRC could also be an agent of his/her institution (e.g., hospital, medical school, and research institute).

Any actions performed improperly during the course of a clinical trial that result in liability might cause the CRC, the PI, or the institution of employment to be liable.

A PI who does not properly supervise those to whom he/she delegates tasks, resulting in harm to the patient, may also be liable.

There are professionals who think that the one with the most money is the one who is sued. This is not true! The fact that a CRC is not a "deep pocket" will not protect him/her from being named in a lawsuit!

XIV. Writing the Study Summary

A vast amount of information is collected during the course of a controlled clinical study. To transform this raw data into useful information, the Sponsor will subject the data to rigorous analyses. The following are typical of the analyses and presentations prepared by the Sponsor.

A. Biostatistical Report

Following the statistical analysis of the data collected during the study, comprehensive computer-generated tabulations are prepared to summarize the trends and changes that occurred. An interpretation of these statistical results is provided in the biostatistical report, which is typically written by a biostatistician.

B. Integrated Clinical Study Report

To present the results of the study to the FDA and other regulatory agencies around the world, the Sponsor will prepare a report that provides a detailed description of the methods, results, and conclusions drawn from the study. This report integrates the key aspects of the biostatistical report with clinical interpretations of the study results. In this manner, a comprehensive overview of the study is prepared for future reference.

C. Articles for Publication

The results of key studies are often written up for submission to scientific journals. The PI or subinvestigators may be given the opportunity to draft the manuscript based on data contained in the Integrated Clinical Study Report. The Sponsor may offer technical or editorial assistance in preparing these articles. Alternatively, data from a study may be presented as an abstract or poster at a scientific meeting.

XV. Achieving Credibility and Recognition as a Clinical Research Coordinator

Achieving credibility and recognition as a CRC in the pharmaceutical industry is not an easy undertaking. To be successful in the pharmaceutical research industry, it is essential to be seen as competent, believable, and confident by the study subjects, CRAs, Sponsors, and other allied health care professionals.

There are several important ways to enhance your credibility as a research professional:

✔ Continually radiate a professional image.

✔ Demonstrate your integrity.

✔ Build good professional relationships.

✔ Be prepared for a monitoring visit.

✔ Ensure a working knowledge of the study and therapeutic area.

In addition, presenting a professional relationship utilizing written correspondence can be achieved in many ways:

✔ Follow a business letter format.

✔ Use letterhead and include the name of the study about which you are writing.

✔ Do not write personal comments or opinions in study-related correspondence.

✔ Remember that people you have never met may review anything you write. It may become a permanent part of a study's regulatory file.

✔ Use spell check and remember to proofread everything to ensure you are using the correct words (i.e., "principal" investigator versus "principle" investigator).

✔ Save personal comments for a time when you are speaking person-to-person.

✔ Print/date and initial study specific emails.

✔ Ensure Notes to File (NTF) prepared by the study staff have the name of the institution, the study title, or at the very least the Protocol number, and that they are dated and signed by the person preparing the NTF. It is a good idea for the PI to, at a minimum, initial the NTF indicating not only agreement with the content but knowledge of the NTF.

✔ Whenever possible use bullet points instead of paragraphs, if appropriate.

Presenting a professional image utilizing voice mail can also be achieved by the following suggestions:

- ✔ Generally, the same rules apply to voice and written correspondence. It may seem redundant, but it is true.

- ✔ Remember that voice-messaging systems can be an open forum, as your message can be forwarded to multiple people.

- ✔ Take a moment and make sure you are leaving a message for the correct person at his/her extension. If you inadvertently leave a voice mail message on the wrong extension, the message may take on a *"life of its own,"* as it is forwarded companywide until/if the message reaches the person for whom it was intended.

- ✔ Messages should be *short* and to the point.

- ✔ Briefly indicate the reason why you are calling. This will better enable the CRA to quickly respond to your needs.

- ✔ If the CRA is on vacation or not available, in most cases you would be directed to contact a study manager in the CRA's absence. When a CRA is not in his/her office, in most cases, the company requires the CRA to utilize the "Out of Office Assistant" indicating he/she is out of the office and when he/she will return. In many cases a cell phone number is noted if the CRA needs to be contacted immediately.

- ✔ Remember to document the conversation in a Telephone Contact Report (TCR). Do not forget to print/date and initial the TCR and file the TCR in the correspondence section of the Site Regulatory Binder. Unless you have been instructed otherwise, you do not need to document the CRA's confirmation of a study-related visit. Utilizing a visit confirmation letter can serve the same purpose as a TCR while saving paper.

- ✔ Provide the CRA with a copy of the TRC for placement in the Master File for your site.

Presenting a professional image utilizing email can be achieved in many ways:

- ✔ Email messaging can be an open forum because your message, even if it is bcc (blind carbon copied) and marked "confidential," can be forwarded to multiple people.

- ✔ Make sure you are sending the email to the correct email address.

- ✔ Make sure when you respond to an email sent to the entire study team, including sites, you respond only to the name of the person sending the email. If you reply to all you may find your response has been sent to the entire email listing.

✔ Do not forward the following types of email messages:

    ✔ Chain emails, including political emails and jokes (something you think is funny may be offensive to another).

    ✔ Emails using profanity or anything not related to the study.

✔ Do not put your favorite CRA on any kind of email mailing list. Sponsors may periodically monitor their employees' email messages.

Demonstrating your integrity can be achieved via the following ways:

✔ Make sure you keep commitments.

✔ Let the CRA know if you are not going to be ready for his/her visit. Do not call a CRA at the last minute (some CRAs have actually been called at the airport while they were getting ready to travel to the site). Provide the CRA enough time so that the visit can be rescheduled.

✔ Rescheduling a previously scheduled visit for one study to accommodate a visit for another study is not appropriate, nor is it fair to the CRA's site visit schedule.

✔ Understand mistakes are made by everyone, including the CRA, and successful research Protocol is a team effort. The mistake is not as important as the methods used to correct the mistake and ensure policies, training, etc., to ensure the same mistakes do not occur in the future.

✔ During a monitoring visit, when additional clarification or deviations are noted, remember the CRA is only doing his/her job. You or your site are not being singled out. The only reason the CRA brings these to your attention is to ensure the study is being conducted according to the Protocol specifics.

✔ Don't take on more work than you can realistically handle. While it is understood that in many cases this is not something within your control, being prepared for a specific visit is important to meet project-specific time lines.

✔ Be careful not to speak negatively about another professional. You never know if there is someone present, or within listening distance, who knows of the individual about whom you are speaking and the conversation could be repeated. Regardless, if the Sponsor representative or the CRA makes negative remarks about another site, do not fall into the trap of being part of the conversation.

A. Attending Investigator Meetings

Investigator Meetings generally take place in a specific geographical area convenient for all sites participating in the Protocol. During an Investigator Meeting all aspects of the Protocol are discussed. This is an opportunity for those attending the Investigator Meeting to ask questions, provide suggestions, and share information with other participating sites.

When attending an Investigator Meeting, the following is important in achieving credibility:

✔ Be on time for all training sessions. Tardiness is always noted by the Sponsor and the Sponsor representatives.

✔ Turn off your cell phone, as this can be a distraction not only to the person presenting but to the attendees as well.

✔ During the training sessions, constantly going in and out of the session can be a distraction to not only the person presenting but to the attendees as well. There will be instances when you must leave the training session. In these instances, return to the session as soon as possible.

✔ Not attending a training session to sightsee or shop is not appropriate. All absences are noted by the Sponsor and the Sponsor representatives and will reflect negatively on your site. This includes going with the PI.

✔ Spending a lot of time at the hotel bar drinking will not add to your credibility and will raise questions in the minds of the Sponsor and Sponsor representatives.

✔ Do not become inebriated during the cocktail reception or after the dinner; this includes going out to a club after dinner.

✔ Do not discuss the quality or quantity of the food with other attendees. The Sponsor or the Sponsor representative might overhear your comments.

✔ Dress professionally. You are representing your site at this meeting and inappropriate dress will be noted by the Sponsor and the Sponsor representatives.

Remember, the primary purpose of the Investigator Meeting is to discuss the Protocol and to learn how to perform Protocol-specific assessments.

B. How to Work With a Difficult Clinical Research Associate

First, remember the CRA is there to assist you in the successful completion of the clinical trial. It's possible you might not agree with his/her findings or method of monitoring (every CRA has developed their own system of monitoring). The following are suggestions for dealing with some specific problems encountered between the CRA and the CRC:

✔ The CRA is consistently late for scheduled monitoring visits (this does not include airline delays or traffic delays). Discuss how this consistent tardiness impacts your schedule.

✔ The CRA is not dressed professionally. Explain to the CRA how you expect the CRA to be dressed when conducting a monitoring visit at your site.

✔ The CRA constantly makes negative remarks about other sites working on the same Protocol. Explain to the CRA that these comments are not appropriate and remind him/her these are confidentiality issues and should not be discussed.

✔ You may have a policy at your site regarding the CRA wearing perfume/cologne due to allergies with employees or patients. If your site has this policy, let the CRA know at the time the first visit is scheduled, and don't wait until the CRA has been to the site several times. Once informed, if the CRA ignores this policy, explain why it is important. It would also be a good idea to post a sign in the reception areas, as this would apply to patients as well.

✔ If a CRA is confrontational and disrespectful, communicate with the CRA how this behavior is not productive.

Communication is the key to working with a difficult CRA. If the problems persist, and you have discussed these with the CRA, then contact the Project Manager for the Protocol and explain your concerns. Perhaps a three-way conversation amongst you, the CRA, and the Project Manager would resolve these issues. Requesting another CRA as the monitor for your site might not always be the solution, and you may find it will require more time from your schedule to become familiar with the new CRA and his/her style of monitoring. Remember, this goes both ways. If a Study Coordinator is difficult to work with, the CRA will discuss this with you personally before discussing your actions with the PI. There should never be a "power struggle" between the CRA and the Study Coordinator. The successful completion of a clinical trial can only be accomplished by a team effort. This cannot be stressed enough.

XVI. Electronic Data Capture and Clinical Trials

The collection of data obtained during a clinical trial historically has been a manual, labor-intensive paper-based process. Information is generated from the Protocol-specific assessments, which are recorded in the patient's medical record as well as the Protocol-related subject study binder or workfolder. This information is then manually recorded on a paper CRF by the Study Coordinator or a data coordinator. The completion of CRFs by data coordinators is rapidly replacing the task once primarily performed by CRCs. The increasing duties of CRCs, the size of facilities and the number of Protocols being conducted, and in many cases, the actual paper CRF not being completed in a timely fashion are the reasons for this change.

In response, several companies have been created to provide investigative sites with data coordinators for the sole purpose of completing the paper CRFs. Many institutions, realizing there is a need for personnel to transcribe the information from the source documents onto the paper CRF, have provided for trained clerical personnel to complete this task rather than the CRC.

Periodically, during the conduct of the Protocol, a CRA from the sponsoring pharmaceutical company will perform a monitoring visit. One purpose of the monitoring visit is to ensure the Protocol-specific assessments have been completed according to the Protocol guidelines and to review the data contained in the source documents to ensure the information in the CRF is consistent with the information in the source documents. During the review of the study specific information, inconsistencies and/or corrections are noted on "monitoring notes," which are discussed with the Research Study Coordinator, and then corrections are completed.

Once the CRFs have been retrieved by the CRA and sent to Data Management, the data are then manually entered into a Central Data Management System (CDMS). When inconsistencies are noted, or further clarification is needed, the Data Clarification Forms (DCFs) are generated to address the inconsistencies or additional clarification. It seems there are always a fair number of DCFs requiring attention by the CRC and/or PI. Even though the CRC or the PI may not have completed the CRF, they are responsible for the information contained in the source documents that were transcribed on the CRF. The process is labor-intensive, slow, and archaic, considering we live in a technically advanced society.

According to David Handelsman, "Few industries are considered to be as cutting-edge as the life sciences industries. The advancement in drug development and biomedical devices are often astonishing and can sometimes seem like something straight out of an old movie. But the reality is that some of the underlying technologies and business processes are more like an old silent motion picture. One area that has been particularly slow in catching up with the electronic age is the capturing of information for use in clinical trials." During the past 20 years, technology has been developed to assist in electronically capturing clinical trials data. Although electronic data capture (EDC) is not a new concept, pharmaceutical companies have taken a long time to widely adopt this concept in the conduct of clinical trials. There are, however, organizations that have begun to recognize the value of using EDC. If you attend a medical conference, you cannot avoid the showcase of the various EDC products on display.

The term "electronic data capture" encompasses several different types of technology used in the conduct of clinical research. EDC can be defined as:

- ✔ electronic replacement for paper CRFs; or
- ✔ interactive voice response system, which is used in the conduct of clinical trials by following voice prompts developed specifically for each Protocol. This is a telephone interactive system used to:
  - ✔ randomize a subject to a specific Protocol treatment;
  - ✔ dispense investigational products (IP) to a subject during participation in a trial;
  - ✔ acknowledge receipt of the IP at the investigational site;
  - ✔ report subject visits; and
  - ✔ report information via telephone or even by PDA, such as a BlackBerry or similar device, for information obtained by home during their participation in a clinical trial.

Regardless of the type of EDC, the intent is the same: to replace the paper-based process of capturing information with an electronic system to expedite the availability of accurate data for the clinical trial.

Pharmaceutical companies that use EDC programs can obtain clinical data quickly, frequently, and accurately, while omitting paper-based forms. This also allows the CRA, as well as the investigational sites using an EDC system, to replace the need for manually collecting and entering the information. Validation of data with the EDC system is quicker and is designed to prompt the person entering the data when there is inconsistent or inaccurate data. For example, if a birth date 10 Feb 79 is entered as 10 Feb 2009, the system queries the date immediately, so it can be corrected before the data ever leaves the Investigator's office. This instant validation process provides a much higher level of data quality at a reduced cost, while maintaining the integrity of the information entered into the EDC system.

Most pharmaceutical companies have realized the benefits of EDC and have begun to develop their own EDC systems, while also utilizing existing EDC systems. Depending on the type of programs in use, either completely EDC-oriented or only partially electronic, a CRC may have to work on two different Protocols from one pharmaceutical company using two different EDC programs. If an investigational site works on several Protocols with several Sponsors, there may also be other EDC systems. This can present a problem for the site's staff as it takes time for the staff as well as the CRA to learn each program. The ideal situation would be for the various EDC vendors to have a standardized methodology. Capturing clinical data is one of the critical components of their business and the benefits are significant. As a result, as mentioned previously, many pharmaceutical companies work with multiple EDC vendors, and in many cases have developed their own EDC systems.

There is a growing interest in having pharmaceutical companies adopt a common data collection format. The common format could significantly elevate the strain on both the clinical research site staff as well as the research sites typically working with multiple Sponsors on multiple studies. It is inefficient if every study uses a different EDC. At some point it is likely the ECD vendors will consolidate, making it easier for pharmaceutical companies to select a vendor and for the site staff to become proficient with a limited number of EDC Systems.

There is also a growing interest in the pharmaceutical industries to adopt a common data collection format. This common format would significantly ease the burden on both the research sites and pharmaceutical companies. The growing adoption of Clinical Data Interchange Standards Consortium (CDISC) recommended, common methodology is likely to spearhead this effort. The CDISC data standards and data models can be applied to the design of data capture screens so that EDC interfaces are similar between products. At a broader level, the Protocol representation group within CDISC is providing common methods to define the Protocol or the rules of conduct for a research Protocol. For example, data-related activities associated with a clinical trial can be defined in the same context as the rules. This will further expedite automatic data collection, data management, and analysis.

There are other obstacles facing pharmaceutical companies utilizing ECD:

✔ What should be done with the EDC information as it is collected?

✔ Where should it be stored?

✔ Should it be put back into the paper-based CDMS?

✔ Should it be made available in an analytical system?

EDC, as successful as it may be, is not the only source of data available for use in clinical trials. Data also come from sources such as the clinical laboratory, reading centers for specific Protocol procedures, and CROs.

There are still many unanswered questions regarding the collection of data in an EDC system and how to integrate and manage the EDC data with the other data so that pharmaceutical companies can make accurate and timely scientific decisions.

Many pharmaceutical companies are beginning to entirely phase out their CDMS, or the paper-based CRF system. They recognize that the cost incurred to use this type of system is no longer necessary. These organizations are focused on an EDC philosophy and are using a repository, such as SAS Drug Development, for storing and managing the EDC and other associated data in order to make it readily available for analysis and integration.

In an effort to help pharmaceutical companies accelerate the transition to ECD, SAS has established partnerships with several leading EDC vendors such as Phase Forward, Oracle, DATATRAK, and etrials. The goal is to conduct clinical trials in timely manner, with the necessary documentation readily accessible, and ultimately to support the primary goal of providing safe and effective drugs to market faster.

As the EDC market matures and more organizations begin to experience the benefits of EDC, the use of EDC will become the standard method of conducting clinical research.

XVII. Appendices

APPENDIX I: Helpful Sources

A. Names and Addresses of Clinical Research Resources

Membership Organizations

ACRP (Association of Clinical Research Professionals)
500 Montgomery Street
Suite# 800
Alexandria, VA 22314
Telephone: 703-254-8100
Fax: 703-254-8101
Email: office@acrpnet.org
Website: www.acrpnet.org
ACRP also has affiliate offices in each state. Contact the main ACRP office for the location in your state.

American Society of Law, Medicine & Ethics
765 Commonwealth Avenue
Suite# 1634
Boston, MA 02215
Telephone: 617-262-4990
Fax: 617-437-7596
Website: www.aslme.org

DIA (Drug Information Association)
800 Enterprise Road
Suite #200
Horsham, PA 19044-3594
Telephone: 215-442-6100
Fax: 215-442-6199
Email: dia@diahome.org
Website: www.diahome.org

PRIM&R (Public Responsibility in Medicine and Research)
126 Brookline Avenue
Suite #202
Boston, MA 02215-3920
Telephone: 617-423-4112

Fax: 617-423-1185
Website: www.primr.org
PRIM&R's Executive Office is also the Administrative Site for ARENA (Applied Research Ethics National Association).

Legal Services

Francis X. Sexton, Jr., Esq.
355 Alhambra Circle
Suite # 1250
Coral Gables, FL 33134
Telephone: 305-444-6669
Email: fsexton@cfclaw.com

Commercial IRBs (Central IRBs)

Health Industry Manufacturers Association (HIMA)
1200 G. Street NW
Suite #400
Washington, DC 20005-3814
Telephone: 202-783-8700
Fax: 202-783-8750
Website: www.himanet.com
For a complete listing of all commercial IRBs, contact HIMA.

Publications

Ethics and Regulations of Clinical Research, by Robert J. Levine
2nd Edition, 1988, Paperback
This edition is out of print, but copies can be found on the web.

Glossary of Lay Language Synonyms, for Common Terms Used in Informed Consent Documents for Clinical Studies: A Handbook for Clinical Researchers, by Deborrah Norris
1996, Paperback
Plexus Publishing, Inc., www.plexuspublishing.com

Seminars/Workshops

Contact the following organizations directly for information:

ACRP (Association of Clinical Research Professionals)
Telephone: 202-737-8100
Website: www.acrpnet.org

American Society of Phlebotomy Technicians
Website: www.aspt.org

American Society of Law, Medicine & Ethics
Telephone: 617-262-4990
Website: www.aslme.org

DIA (Drug Information Association)
Telephone: 215-628-2288
Website: www.diahome.org

FDA (U.S. Food and Drug Administration)
Telephone: 301-443-2894
Website: www.fda.gov

HAZMAT Certification
Website: www.hazmatschool.com

Lucy Vanpelt, PA (Clinical Research Study Coordinators Specific Training and Onsite Training)
Telephone: 954-923-5909
Email: dlucyvanpelt@aol.com

NIH Certification
Website: phrp.nihtraining.com/uses/login/php
No cost, web-based.

PRIM&R/ARENA
Telephone: 617-423-4112
Website: www.primr.org

University of Miami—CITI
Website: www.citiprogram.org
University-based but can be taken as an individual; not associated with University of Miami.

WIRB (Western Institutional Review Board)
Telephone: 360-754-9248
Website: www.wirb.com

B. Important FDA Websites for Institutional Review Boards and Clinical Investigators

Check out the following websites, which both contain information that is pertinent to your role in conducting clinical research:

- FDA Guidances We Develop and Enforcement Information
  (www.fda.gov/CDER/regulatory/default.htm)

- FDA.com: Food and Drug Assistance, Resources for Industry and Consumers (www.fda.com)

APPENDIX II: Forms Used During the Course of a Clinical Study

Form 1. Information Regarding Participation in a Clinical Trial

This form can be used to develop a handout to provide potential subjects with information regarding their expectations when considering participating in a clinical trial. These handouts are not study specific and contain your site's information:

- ✔ Name of institution/clinic
- ✔ Address of institution/clinic including phone number
- ✔ Logo if used on letterhead, etc.

What Is a Clinical Trial?

A clinical trial is a research study conducted to evaluate the safety and effectiveness of a new Investigational Product (medications or devices) not yet available to the public, or an Investigational Product (medications or devices) available to the public. A clinical trial must adhere to the strict regulatory guidelines established by the Food and Drug Administration (FDA) and other regulatory agencies. *Participation in a clinical trial is voluntary.* Your physician may suggest benefits from participating in a clinical trial; however, the decision to volunteer *is yours alone to make.*

Most clinical trials are conducted in phases. There are four main phases of clinical trials:

- ✔ Phase I
- ✔ Phase II
- ✔ Phase III
- ✔ Phase IV

Phase I clinical trials help to establish not only the safest dose of an Investigational Product but the overall safety of the Investigational Product being tested, which is of utmost importance. These clinical trials are generally conducted in a small number of healthy volunteers, both men and women, with no critical medical conditions, including the condition the drug or device is being tested for. In many cases, a Phase I clinical trial is the first time the Investigational Product (medications or devices) is being used in people.

Phase II clinical trials help to establish that the appropriate doses determined in the Phase I clinical trial are safe as well as effective. These clinical trials are generally conducted in a larger number of volunteers of both men and women who have the specific medical condition the Investigational Product is being developed to treat.

Phase III clinical trials help to confirm the doses of the Investigational Product are safe and effective for the medical treatment the Investigational Product is being tested for. The number of volunteers for Phase III clinical trials can range from 100 to 5,000 and may be conducted worldwide.

Phase IV clinical trials are generally performed after the Investigational Product has been approved by the FDA and may provide additional information regarding the Investigational Product to ensure the safety and effectiveness of the Investigational Product.

REMEMBER, DURING ALL PHASES OF A CLINICAL TRIAL, SAFETY OF THE STUDY PARTICIPANT IS MOST IMPORTANT!

Why Do People Volunteer to Participate in a Clinical Trial?

People volunteer to participate in a clinical trial for various reasons:

✔ To receive the latest, most advanced Investigational Product long before the Investigational Product is available to the general public.

✔ To have a medical option to their current medical treatment which may not be effective. It is important to remember that a clinical trial is used specifically for the development an Investigational Product not necessarily to treat your disease.

What Can You Expect if You Volunteer to Participate in a Clinical Trial?

✔ A full medical evaluation and diagnosis made by a qualified physician.

✔ Close medical monitoring, including study related laboratory tests, x-rays, and other medical procedures specific to the clinical trial you volunteer to participate in.

✔ Regular medical examinations to evaluate your progress.

✔ Regular communication with the study staff.

Your participation as a volunteer in a clinical trial begins after you have signed the informed consent, which has been approved by an Institutional Review Board (IRB), whose primary purpose is the protection of human volunteers, such as yourself.

An informed consent is a document that must be approved by an IRB before it can be presented to a potential volunteer. When all your questions and concerns have been addressed by the physician in charge of the clinical trial, and you have had time to review the informed consent document, you will sign the informed consent and your participation in the clinical trial may begin. A copy of the signed informed consent will be provided to you for your records. *Remember, no clinical trial medical procedures, including being asked to stop taking any prescription medications you are taking, can be done until after you have signed the informed consent.*

Participation in a clinical trial is voluntary—you have the right to withdraw your consent at any time during your participation in the clinical trial without any negative effects related to your medical care.

How Does Volunteering for a Clinical Trial Affect Care Received from Your Primary Care Physician?

Your participation in a clinical trial will not affect the care you are receiving from your primary care physician. You are encouraged to talk to your doctor about your participation in a clinical trial. The physician in charge of the clinical trial does not replace your primary care physician but works with your physician to provide you with additional health care options. Your records during your participation in a clinical trial may be shared with our physician, or they may remain confidential at your request.

Participation in a clinical trial is a commitment between you and the physician in charge of the clinical trial. It is important for your own safety and well-being that you follow the instructions given by the research staff, keep all appointments required for the clinical trial, and take the Investigational Product as instructed.

It may be helpful to know your participation in a clinical trial may help in the development of a new Investigational Product, which could benefit many people suffering from the same medical condition.

Form 2. The Statement of Investigator (FDA FORM 1572)

<table>
<tr>
<td colspan="2">DEPARTMENT OF HEALTH AND HUMAN SERVICES
FOOD AND DRUG ADMINISTRATION

STATEMENT OF INVESTIGATOR
(TITLE 21, CODE OF FEDERAL REGULATIONS (CFR) PART 312)
(See instructions on reverse side.)</td>
<td>Form Approved: OMB No. 0910-0014.
Expiration Date: May 31, 2009.
See OMB Statement on Reverse.

NOTE: No investigator may participate in an investigation until he/she provides the sponsor with a completed, signed Statement of Investigator, Form FDA 1572 (21 CFR 312.53(c)).</td>
</tr>
</table>

1. NAME AND ADDRESS OF INVESTIGATOR

2. EDUCATION, TRAINING, AND EXPERIENCE THAT QUALIFIES THE INVESTIGATOR AS AN EXPERT IN THE CLINICAL INVESTIGATION OF THE DRUG FOR THE USE UNDER INVESTIGATION. ONE OF THE FOLLOWING IS ATTACHED.

    ☐ CURRICULUM VITAE   ☐ OTHER STATEMENT OF QUALIFICATIONS

3. NAME AND ADDRESS OF ANY MEDICAL SCHOOL, HOSPITAL OR OTHER RESEARCH FACILITY WHERE THE CLINICAL INVESTIGATION(S) WILL BE CONDUCTED.

4. NAME AND ADDRESS OF ANY CLINICAL LABORATORY FACILITIES TO BE USED IN THE STUDY.

5. NAME AND ADDRESS OF THE INSTITUTIONAL REVIEW BOARD (IRB) THAT IS RESPONSIBLE FOR REVIEW AND APPROVAL OF THE STUDY(IES).

6. NAMES OF THE SUBINVESTIGATORS *(e.g., research fellows, residents, associates)* WHO WILL BE ASSISTING THE INVESTIGATOR IN THE CONDUCT OF THE INVESTIGATION(S).

7. NAME AND CODE NUMBER, IF ANY, OF THE PROTOCOL(S) IN THE IND FOR THE STUDY(IES) TO BE CONDUCTED BY THE INVESTIGATOR.

8. ATTACH THE FOLLOWING CLINICAL PROTOCOL INFORMATION:

☐   FOR PHASE 1 INVESTIGATIONS, A GENERAL OUTLINE OF THE PLANNED INVESTIGATION INCLUDING THE ESTIMATED DURATION OF THE STUDY AND THE MAXIMUM NUMBER OF SUBJECTS THAT WILL BE INVOLVED.

☐   FOR PHASE 2 OR 3 INVESTIGATIONS, AN OUTLINE OF THE STUDY PROTOCOL INCLUDING AN APPROXIMATION OF THE NUMBER OF SUBJECTS TO BE TREATED WITH THE DRUG AND THE NUMBER TO BE EMPLOYED AS CONTROLS, IF ANY; THE CLINICAL USES TO BE INVESTIGATED; CHARACTERISTICS OF SUBJECTS BY AGE, SEX, AND CONDITION; THE KIND OF CLINICAL OBSERVATIONS AND LABORATORY TESTS TO BE CONDUCTED; THE ESTIMATED DURATION OF THE STUDY; AND COPIES OR A DESCRIPTION OF CASE REPORT FORMS TO BE USED.

9. COMMITMENTS:

I agree to conduct the study(ies) in accordance with the relevant, current protocol(s) and will only make changes in a protocol after notifying the sponsor, except when necessary to protect the safety, rights, or welfare of subjects.

I agree to personally conduct or supervise the described investigation(s).

I agree to inform any patients, or any persons used as controls, that the drugs are being used for investigational purposes and I will ensure that the requirements relating to obtaining informed consent in 21 CFR Part 50 and institutional review board (IRB) review and approval in 21 CFR Part 56 are met.

I agree to report to the sponsor adverse experiences that occur in the course of the investigation(s) in accordance with 21 CFR 312.64.

I have read and understand the information in the investigator's brochure, including the potential risks and side effects of the drug.

I agree to ensure that all associates, colleagues, and employees assisting in the conduct of the study(ies) are informed about their obligations in meeting the above commitments.

I agree to maintain adequate and accurate records in accordance with 21 CFR 312.62 and to make those records available for inspection in accordance with 21 CFR 312.68.

I will ensure that an IRB that complies with the requirements of 21 CFR Part 56 will be responsible for the initial and continuing review and approval of the clinical investigation. I also agree to promptly report to the IRB all changes in the research activity and all unanticipated problems involving risks to human subjects or others. Additionally, I will not make any changes in the research without IRB approval, except where necessary to eliminate apparent immediate hazards to human subjects.

I agree to comply with all other requirements regarding the obligations of clinical investigators and all other pertinent requirements in 21 CFR Part 312.

INSTRUCTIONS FOR COMPLETING FORM FDA 1572
STATEMENT OF INVESTIGATOR:

1. Complete all sections. Attach a separate page if additional space is needed.

2. Attach curriculum vitae or other statement of qualifications as described in Section 2.

3. Attach protocol outline as described in Section 8.

4. Sign and date below.

5. FORWARD THE COMPLETED FORM AND ATTACHMENTS TO THE SPONSOR. The sponsor will incorporate this information along with other technical data into an Investigational New Drug Application (IND). INVESTIGATORS SHOULD NOT SEND THIS FORM DIRECTLY TO THE FOOD AND DRUG ADMINISTRATION.

10. SIGNATURE OF INVESTIGATOR	11. DATE

(**WARNING:** A willfully false statement is a criminal offense. U.S.C. Title 18, Sec. 1001.)

FORM FDA 1572 (5/06)   PREVIOUS EDITION IS OBSOLETE.   PAGE 2 OF 2

Example of Form 2, FDA 1572, Completed

DEPARTMENT OF HEALTH AND HUMAN SERVICES FOOD AND DRUG ADMINISTRATION **STATEMENT OF INVESTIGATOR** *(TITLE 21, CODE OF FEDERAL REGULATIONS (CFR) PART 312)* (See instructions on reverse side.)	Form Approved: OMB No. 0910-0014. Expiration Date: May 31, 2009. *See OMB Statement on Reverse.*
	NOTE: No investigator may participate in an investigation until he/she provides the sponsor with a completed, signed Statement of Investigator, Form FDA 1572 (21 CFR 312.53(c)).

1. NAME AND ADDRESS OF INVESTIGATOR
Name of Principal Investigator Conductintg the Study
Include the name and address of facility where the protoocl is being conducted

2. EDUCATION, TRAINING, AND EXPERIENCE THAT QUALIFIES THE INVESTIGATOR AS AN EXPERT IN THE CLINICAL INVESTIGATION OF THE DRUG FOR THE USE UNDER INVESTIGATION. ONE OF THE FOLLOWING IS ATTACHED.

☒ CURRICULUM VITAE   ☐ OTHER STATEMENT OF QUALIFICATIONS

3. NAME AND ADDRESS OF ANY MEDICAL SCHOOL, HOSPITAL OR OTHER RESEARCH FACILITY WHERE THE CLINICAL INVESTIGATION(S) WILL BE CONDUCTED.

Important: List the names and addresses of any facility that will be be evaluating or performing protoocl specific assessemnts on a subject.

ABC Research Centers of America	Clinic Sattalite Office(s)
1234 South Park Road	4234 West 50th Avenue
Anytown, USA	Anytown, USA

4. NAME AND ADDRESS OF ANY CLINICAL LABORATORY FACILITIES TO BE USED IN THE STUDY.
Improtant: List the names and addresses of each labortory processing laboratory examples including a local lab, of applicable when using several different labs, (PK lab). Include the name and address of any facility reviewing study specific ECGs and CT scans, if applicable

Central Research Laboratory	Radiology Associates
1254 South Park Road	5425 SE Avenue
Anytown, USA	Anytown, USA

5. NAME AND ADDRESS OF THE INSTITUTIONAL REVIEW BOARD (IRB) THAT IS RESPONSIBLE FOR REVIEW AND APPROVAL OF THE STUDY(IES).
Institutional Review Board of Anytown
4555 outh West 10th Street
Anytown, USA

If the Sponsor has contracted with a central IRB, you are not obligaged to use the Central IRB if you have a local IRB. Check with the local to see if their meeting schedule will accommodate the Sponsor's timelines. If you have a hospital IRB, and you will use a Central IRB the local IRB will need to provide a Waiver Letter for the Sponsor.

6. NAMES OF THE SUBINVESTIGATORS (*e.g., research fellows, residents, associates*) WHO WILL BE ASSISTING THE INVESTIGATOR IN THE CONDUCT OF THE INVESTIGATION(S).
List all subinvestigators in this section. Check with the Sponsor for direction on which study personnel should be listed on the FDA 1572, ie; research pharmacisit

John Allen, MD
Caroline Paden, MD
Marc Smith, DO
Sally Bell, RN, CRC, CCRC
Michael Sams, Phar. D

When study personnel change, ie: no longer working on the study, or no longer working on the study, the FDA Form 1572 should be revised. Discuss specifics for revising the FDA Form 1572 with the Sponsor or the Sponsor Representative.

7. NAME AND CODE NUMBER, IF ANY, OF THE PROTOCOL(S) IN THE IND FOR THE STUDY(IES) TO BE CONDUCTED BY THE INVESTIGATOR.
Make sure you list the complete title of the protocol, include the IND # if available

Note: If the Sponsor provides the Form FDA 1572 on a computer disc, make sure you print the form out on ONE page, not two pages.

FORM FDA 1572 (5/06)	PREVIOUS EDITION IS OBSOLETE.	PAGE 1 OF 3

8. ATTACH THE FOLLOWING CLINICAL PROTOCOL INFORMATION:

☒ FOR PHASE 1 INVESTIGATIONS, A GENERAL OUTLINE OF THE PLANNED INVESTIGATION INCLUDING THE ESTIMATED DURATION OF THE STUDY AND THE MAXIMUM NUMBER OF SUBJECTS THAT WILL BE INVOLVED.

☐ FOR PHASE 2 OR 3 INVESTIGATIONS, AN OUTLINE OF THE STUDY PROTOCOL INCLUDING AN APPROXIMATION OF THE NUMBER OF SUBJECTS TO BE TREATED WITH THE DRUG AND THE NUMBER TO BE EMPLOYED AS CONTROLS, IF ANY; THE CLINICAL USES TO BE INVESTIGATED; CHARACTERISTICS OF SUBJECTS BY AGE, SEX, AND CONDITION; THE KIND OF CLINICAL OBSERVATIONS AND LABORATORY TESTS TO BE CONDUCTED; THE ESTIMATED DURATION OF THE STUDY; AND COPIES OR A DESCRIPTION OF CASE REPORT FORMS TO BE USED.

9. COMMITMENTS:

I agree to conduct the study(ies) in accordance with the relevant, current protocol(s) and will only make changes in a protocol after notifying the sponsor, except when necessary to protect the safety, rights, or welfare of subjects.

I agree to personally conduct or supervise the described investigation(s).

I agree to inform any patients, or any persons used as controls, that the drugs are being used for investigational purposes and I will ensure that the requirements relating to obtaining informed consent in 21 CFR Part 50 and institutional review board (IRB) review and approval in 21 CFR Part 56 are met.

I agree to report to the sponsor adverse experiences that occur in the course of the investigation(s) in accordance with 21 CFR 312.64.

I have read and understand the information in the investigator's brochure, including the potential risks and side effects of the drug.

I agree to ensure that all associates, colleagues, and employees assisting in the conduct of the study(ies) are informed about their obligations in meeting the above commitments.

I agree to maintain adequate and accurate records in accordance with 21 CFR 312.62 and to make those records available for inspection in accordance with 21 CFR 312.68.

I will ensure that an IRB that complies with the requirements of 21 CFR Part 56 will be responsible for the initial and continuing review and approval of the clinical investigation. I also agree to promptly report to the IRB all changes in the research activity and all unanticipated problems involving risks to human subjects or others. Additionally, I will not make any changes in the research without IRB approval, except where necessary to eliminate apparent immediate hazards to human subjects.

I agree to comply with all other requirements regarding the obligations of clinical investigators and all other pertinent requirements in 21 CFR Part 312.

INSTRUCTIONS FOR COMPLETING FORM FDA 1572
STATEMENT OF INVESTIGATOR:

1. Complete all sections. Attach a separate page if additional space is needed.

2. Attach curriculum vitae or other statement of qualifications as described in Section 2.

3. Attach protocol outline as described in Section 8.

4. Sign and date below.

5. FORWARD THE COMPLETED FORM AND ATTACHMENTS TO THE SPONSOR. The sponsor will incorporate this information along with other technical data into an Investigational New Drug Application (IND). INVESTIGATORS SHOULD NOT SEND THIS FORM DIRECTLY TO THE FOOD AND DRUG ADMINISTRATION.

10. SIGNATURE OF INVESTIGATOR	11. DATE

(WARNING: A willfully false statement is a criminal offense. U.S.C. Title 18, Sec. 1001.)

Public reporting burden for this collection of information is estimated to average 100 hours per response, including the time for reviewing instructions, searching existing data sources, gathering and maintaining the data needed, and completing reviewing the collection of information. Send comments regarding this burden estimate or any other aspect of this collection of information, including suggestions for reducing this burden to:

Department of Health and Human Services
Food and Drug Administration
Center for Drug Evaluation and Research
Central Document Room
5901-B Ammendale Road
Beltsville, MD 20705-1266

Department of Health and Human Services
Food and Drug Administration
Center for Biologics Evaluation and Research (HFM-99)
1401 Rockville Pike
Rockville, MD 20852-1448

"An agency may not conduct or sponsor, and a person is not required to respond to, a collection of information unless it displays a currently valid OMB control number."

Please DO NOT RETURN this application to this address.

Form 3. Bill of Rights for Study Subject Volunteers

Any study subject volunteer consenting to participate in a clinical trial, or a legally authorized third party who is asked to give his/her consent on behalf of another, has the following rights:

✔ The right to be allowed to ask any questions about the clinical trial before giving consent, as well as during the study subject volunteer's participation in the clinical trial.

✔ The right to be given enough time, without pressure from the research staff, before signing the informed consent document to decide whether to participate in the clinical trial.

✔ The right to receive a copy of the signed and dated informed consent document for participation in the clinical trial.

✔ The right to be told the reason for the clinical trial.

✔ The right to be told the known benefits that can reasonably be expected during participation in the clinical trial.

✔ The right to be told what kinds of medical tests will be done, how many clinical visits there will be, how long the clinical visits will take, and if there are any questionnaires or diary cards that need to be completed during participation in a clinical trial.

✔ The right to be told if there are alternate treatments available to the study subject volunteer.

✔ The right to be told if there are other options available and how these options may be better or worse than participating in the clinical trial.

✔ The right to be told about all the known side effects or discomforts that might reasonably be expected during participation in the clinical trial.

✔ The right to be told of any medical treatments available if any complications occur during participation in the clinical trial.

✔ The right to be told who will be responsible for paying the cost of the medical treatments if any complications occur during participation in the clinical trial.

✔ The right to refuse to participate for any reason, before and during the clinical trial.

✔ The right to be told of any information learned during the clinical trial that might influence he/she.

If you have any questions regarding your rights as a volunteer for a clinical trial, it is VERY important to make sure you discuss these questions with the research staff.

Form 4. The MedWatch Adverse Experience Form

U.S. Department of Health and Human Services

Form Approved: OMB No. 0910-0291, Expires:10/31/08
See OMB statement on reverse.

MEDWATCH

The FDA Safety Information and
Adverse Event Reporting Program

For VOLUNTARY reporting of
adverse events, product problems and
product use errors

General Instructions   Page _____ of _____

FDA USE ONLY

Triage unit
sequence #

A. PATIENT INFORMATION   Section A - Help

1. Patient Identifier	2. Age at Time of Event, or Date of Birth:	3. Sex	4. Weight
In confidence		☐ Female ☐ Male	_____ lb or _____ kg

B. ADVERSE EVENT, PRODUCT PROBLEM OR ERROR

Check all that apply: Section B - Help

1. ☐ Adverse Event   ☐ Product Problem (e.g., defects/malfunctions)
☐ Product Use Error   ☐ Problem with Different Manufacturer of Same Medicine

2. Outcomes Attributed to Adverse Event
(Check all that apply)

☐ Death: _____ (mm/dd/yyyy)   ☐ Disability or Permanent Damage
☐ Life-threatening   ☐ Congenital Anomaly/Birth Defect
☐ Hospitalization - initial or prolonged   ☐ Other Serious (Important Medical Events)
☐ Required Intervention to Prevent Permanent Impairment/Damage (Devices)

3. Date of Event (mm/dd/yyyy)	4. Date of this Report (mm/dd/yyyy) 09/14/2007

5. Describe Event, Problem or Product Use Error

(Continue on page 2)

6. Relevant Tests/Laboratory Data, Including Dates

(Continue on page 2)

7. Other Relevant History, Including Preexisting Medical Conditions (e.g., allergies, race, pregnancy, smoking and alcohol use, liver/kidney problems, etc.)

(Continue on page 2)

C. PRODUCT AVAILABILITY   Section C - Help

Product Available for Evaluation? (Do not send product to FDA)

☐ Yes   ☐ No   ☐ Returned to Manufacturer on: _____ (mm/dd/yyyy)

PLEASE TYPE OR USE BLACK INK

D. SUSPECT PRODUCT(S)   Section D - Help

1. Name, Strength, Manufacturer (from product label)
#1
#2

2.	Dose or Amount	Frequency	Route
#1			
#2			

3. Dates of Use (If unknown, give duration) from/to (or best estimate)	5. Event Abated After Use Stopped or Dose Reduced?
#1	#1 ☐ Yes ☐ No ☐ Doesn't Apply
#2	#2 ☐ Yes ☐ No ☐ Doesn't Apply

4. Diagnosis or Reason for Use (Indication)	8. Event Reappeared After Reintroduction?
#1	#1 ☐ Yes ☐ No ☐ Doesn't Apply
#2	#2 ☐ Yes ☐ No ☐ Doesn't Apply

6. Lot #	7. Expiration Date	
#1	#1	9. NDC # or Unique ID
#2	#2	

E. SUSPECT MEDICAL DEVICE   Section E - Help

1. Brand Name

2. Common Device Name

3. Manufacturer Name, City and State

4. Model #	Lot #	5. Operator of Device
Catalog #	Expiration Date (mm/dd/yyyy)	☐ Health Professional ☐ Lay User/Patient
Serial #	Other #	☐ Other:

6. If Implanted, Give Date (mm/dd/yyyy)	7. If Explanted, Give Date (mm/dd/yyyy)

8. Is this a Single-use Device that was Reprocessed and Reused on a Patient?
☐ Yes   ☐ No

9. If Yes to Item No. 8, Enter Name and Address of Reprocessor

F. OTHER (CONCOMITANT) MEDICAL PRODUCTS   Section F - Help

Product names and therapy dates (exclude treatment of event)

(Continue on page 2)

G. REPORTER   (Confidentiality statement)   Section G - Help

1. Name and Address

Phone #	E-mail

2. Health Professional?	3. Occupation	4. Also Reported to:
☐ Yes ☐ No		☐ Manufacturer

5. If you do NOT want your identity disclosed to the manufacturer, place an "X" in this box: ☐
☐ User Facility
☐ Distributor/Importer

FORM FDA 3500 (10/05)   Submission of a report does not constitute an admission that medical personnel or the product caused or contributed to the event.

Form 5. Informed Consent Form

INFORMED CONSENT   **PROTOCOL ID:**_____

DOCUMENTATION FORM

Mr./Ms. _____was approached by Dr./Mr./Ms._____
regarding his/her interest in the above referenced research protocol. After acknowledging
interest, the potential candidate met with the Principal Investigator/Research Coordinator
_____ to initiate the informed consent. The initial informed consent discussion
lasted _____minutes and consisted of a complete review of the informed consent
documents covering all the essential elements and pertinent additional elements of the informed
consent.

The potential candidate had opportunity to have questions answered to his/her satisfaction. A
copy of the informed consent was given to the potential participant to review and ample time was
given for him/her to decide whether to participate. Copies of the SIGNED informed consent
documents were given to the participant, placed in the medical record and in the research file.

No exculpatory language was used in this discussion, and there was no coercion on the part of
the investigator or the research staff. Any conflict of interest issues have been disclosed in the
informed consent document and discussion.

_____   Date:_____
Signed (Person Obtaining Consent/Evaluator)

_____

Print Name

Attachments:

____Protocol Consent

____HIPAA Consent

____Other_____

INFORMED CONSENT   **PROTOCOL ID:**_____

EVALUATION TO SIGN CONSENT FORM

Subject ID:_____   **Subject Initials:**_____**Date of Rating:**_____

PROCEDURE:

Make a subjective judgment regarding item 1 below. Ask the subject questions 2–5. The evaluator may select the language to use in asking the questions in order to help the subject understand them.

ITEMS: **SCORE:**

1. Is the subject alert and able to communicate with the evaluator? _____   _____
    Yes = 2, No = 0

2. Ask the subject to name at least two (2) potential risks incurred as a result of   _____
    participating in the study. Unable = 0, Lists one = 1, Lists two = 2

    _____

    _____

3. Ask the subject to name at least two (2) things that will be expected of   _____
    him/her in terms of patient cooperation during the study. Unable = 0,
    Lists one = 1, Lists two = 2

    _____

    _____

4. Ask the subject to explain what he/she would do if he/she decides to no   _____
    longer participate in the study. Unable = 0, Answers, but not the most
    appropriate response = 1, Talks to any staff member = 2

    _____

5. Ask the subject to explain what he/she would do if he/she were experiencing   _____
    distress or discomfort. Doesn't know = 0, Answers, but not the most
    appropriate response = 1, Talks to any staff member = 2

    _____

SIGNATURES:

I hereby certify that the above subject is alert, able to communicate, and able to   _____
give acceptable answers to items 2, 3, 4 and 5 above.   **TOTAL**

Evaluator/Date:_____

Form 6. The Administrative Checklist

Protocol # _____

Protocol Title _____

_____

Sponsor _____

Test Article _____

Clinical Research Associate _____

Phone # _____ Fax # _____

Email Address _____

Name of Laboratory _____

Phone # _____ Fax # _____

Institutional Review Board (IRB) _____

Chairperson _____

Phone # _____ Fax # _____

Email Address _____

Protocol Approval Date _____ Informed Consent Date _____

Principal Investigator _____

Subinvestigator(s) _____

_____

Study Coordinator _____

Study Initiation Date _____ Investigator Meeting Date _____

Documents on File

__ Form FDA 1572	__ Completed Financial Disclosure Form
__ CVs/Medical License	__ Serious Adverse Event Form
__ Laboratory Certification	__ Laboratory Normals/Values
__ Complete Signed Protocol	__ MedWatch Forms
__ Protocol Signature Page	__ Site Signature Log
__ Protocol Amendments	__ Laboratory Submission Reports
__ IRB Membership Lists	__ Monitor Site Visit Log
__ IRB Approval Letter	__ Informed Consent Approval Letter
__ IRB Approved Informed Consents	__ Telephone Log
__ Original Signed Consents	__ Letter of Indemnification
__ Investigator Brochure	__ Shipping Invoices for ALL Supplies
__ Drug Accountability	__ On-going Correspondence
__ Enrollment Logs	__ Informed Consent Logs
__ Investigator Meeting Agenda	__ Investigator/Meeting Attendee List
__ Confidentiality Agreement	__ Delegation of Responsibilities
__ Miscellaneous Sponsor Forms	__ Other Source Documents

NOTE:

All financial records including the following *SHOULD NOT* be part of the Site Binder and should be kept separate:

- ✔ study budget;
- ✔ signed Study Agreement with financial compensation; and
- ✔ signed Financial Disclosure Form (may be included depending upon Sponsor's SOPs).

However, these can be requested by the FDA during an audit.

Form 7. Initial Adverse Experience Report Sheet

Date _____

Study Protocol # _____

Study Investigator _____

Subject I.D. (initials and #) _____

Date subject entered study _____

If subject discontinued study:

Date drug discontinued _____

Date subject discontinued study _____

Description of adverse experience _____

_____

*Diagnostic procedure(s) performed _____

_____

Relationship to study drug ("not related," "possibly," "definitely") _____

Subject's present condition _____

Was subject hospitalized? _____

Was sponsor notified? _____

Name of sponsor's representative contracted/date contracted _____

*May not be applicable

_____

Clinical Research Coordinator (*signature*)

Form 8. Source Sample Telephone Log

Date _____   Time_____

Conversation With _____

Affiliation _____

Telephone # _____

Regarding (Product, Study #, Subject #) _____

       ❏ I Placed Call   ❏ I Returned Call

       ❏ Party Called   ❏ Party Returned Call

_____

_____

_____

_____

_____

_____

_____

_____

_____

Is action or follow-up necessary?   ❏ No   ❏ Yes (specify) _____

_____

_____

- -

Was action taken?   ❏ No   ❏ Yes (specify) _____

_____

_____

_____

Date filed in study file _____

Signed _____

        cc: _____

            _____

            _____

Form 9. Sample Study Advertisement Office Sign

DO YOU HAVE [*insert study indication here*]?

If you are between the ages of ____ and ____ years, and you have been diagnosed with _____ or have any of the following symptoms on a frequent basis:

_____   _____

_____   _____

_____   _____

_____   _____

_____   _____

_____   _____

[*list signs and symptoms of disease/indication being studied*]

then you may qualify for entry into a medical research program. Please contact a nurse, receptionist, or your doctor for more information regarding this free program.

Note: IRB and Sponsor approval are required before posting signs in public areas.

Form 10. Sample Screen Visit Letter

(*Note: Print on site letterhead stationary*.)

Date:

RE: Protocol #

Dear _____:
This letter is to confirm our conversation regarding your potential participation in the above refer-enced research study being performed at our office. This study will involve people who have a diag-nosis of _____. Your screening visit is scheduled for _____ at _____, with _____.

After you have reviewed the informed consent, had all your questions answered, and have agreed to participate in this clinical trial, you will be required to: (list the study requirements here).
(*Note: It is important that no study-related procedures be performed prior to the signing of the informed consent, e.g., fasting for baseline laboratory samples, wash-out of restricted medications.*)

Your participation in this clinical trial is greatly appreciated. If you have any questions regarding your potential participation in this study, do not hesitate to contact me directly at _____.
I look forward to meeting with you.

Sincerely,

_____
Clinical Research Study Coordinator

Form 11. Sample Baseline Visit Letter

(*Note: Print on site letterhead stationary.*)

Date:

RE: Protocol #

Dear _____:
This letter is to confirm the date and time of your baseline visit for participation in the _____
research study. Your appointment has been scheduled for _____ at _____, with
_____.

During your baseline visit, you will be required to undergo the following study procedures:
(*Note: Some examples of study-related procedures*)

- ✔ complete physical exam;
- ✔ ECG;
- ✔ provide laboratory specimens; and
- ✔ chest radiograph.

In addition, you must fast for at least ___ hours prior to having your blood drawn. This means you
may not have any food or drink (including water) for the given specified time period before your
scheduled appointment. A sample of your urine will be obtained as well.

I look forward to working with you on this research study. If you have any questions about your participation in this research study, please do not hesitate to contact me at _____.

Your participation is greatly appreciated.

Sincerely,

_____
Clinical Research Study Coordinator

Form 12. Ongoing Study Visit Letter

(*Note: Print on site letterhead stationary.*)

Date:

RE: Protocol #

Dear _____:
This letter is to confirm your next clinic visit for the _____ study on _____
at _____, with _____.

During this visit, you will be required to undergo the following study-related procedures:
(*Note: List study-specific procedures here.*)

Should you need to take any medication other than the study medication between your first and subsequent visit, you will be asked to keep a record of the dates, the dosages, and reason for the medication so you may report them to me during your clinical visit. In addition, should you experience any unpleasant side effects, you need to keep a record of what they are, when they started, and how long they lasted so you may also report them to me during your clinic visit.

It is important that you remember to bring with you to this visit all unused study medication, including the box and empty blister packs and study supplies, along with your patient diary (if applicable).

It is extremely important that you keep your scheduled clinic visit. If for some reason you are unable to keep this appointment, kindly contact me immediately so that we can reschedule the appointment according to the study guidelines.

Thank you for your continued participation in this research study. In the meantime, please do not hesitate to contact me at (__)_____ if you have any questions or require additional information.

Sincerely,

_____
Clinical Research Study Coordinator

Form 13. Sample Final Study Letter

Date:

RE: Protocol #

Dear _____:

Dr. _____ and I would like to take this opportunity to express our sincere appreciation for your participation in Protocol _____

_____.

Without participants like you, clinical research would not be possible.

Please do no hesitate to contact me in the future if you have any questions regarding your participation in this research study. Again, thank you for your participation.

Sincerely,

_____

Clinical Research Study Coordinator

_____

Principal Investigator

Form 14. Sample Financial Disclosure Certification Form

Principal Investigator's Name _____

Protocol # _____

Investigational Product _____

IND # _____

With respect to the clinical study for the Investigational Product referenced above that I am conducting for (*insert sponsoring pharmaceutical company's name*), I hereby certify to the truth and accuracy of the following statements in compliance with 21 CFR part 54, with the understanding that I am certifying not only for myself as a clinical investigator, but also for my spouse and for each dependent child of mine:

I certify that:

- ✔ I have not entered into any financial arrangement with (*insert sponsoring pharmaceutical company's name*) (e.g., bonus, royalty, or other financial incentive) whereby the outcome of the clinical study could affect my compensation;

- ✔ I do not have a proprietary interest (e.g., patent, trademark, copyright, licensing agreement, etc.) in the Investigational Product tested in the above referenced clinical study;

- ✔ I do not have a significant equity interest (e.g., any ownership interest, stock option, or other financial interest, the value of which cannot be calculated with reference to publicly available prices) in (*insert sponsoring pharmaceutical company's name*); and

- ✔ I have not received significant payments from (*insert sponsoring pharmaceutical company's name*), on or after February 2, 1999, having a total value in excess of $25,000, other than payments for conducting the clinical study. Examples of such significant payments include, but are not limited to, grants or funding for ongoing research, compensation in the form of equipment, or retainers for ongoing consultation and honoraria that are (a) paid directly to me or to the institution with which I am affiliated, and (b) in support of my activities.

Or

I disclose the following (***check all boxes that apply and attach detailed information***):

- ❏ I have entered into a financial arrangement with (*insert sponsoring pharmaceutical company's name*), whereby the value of my compensation could be influenced by the outcome of the clinical study;

❑ I am receiving significant payments from (*insert sponsoring pharmaceutical company's name*) on or after February 2, 1999, having value in excess of $25,000, other than payment for conducting the above clinical study. Examples of significant payments include, but are not limited to, grants or funding for ongoing research, compensation in the form of equipment, or retainers for ongoing consultation and honoraria that are (a) paid directly to me or to the institution with which I am affiliated, and (b) paid in support of my activities;

❑ I hold a proprietary interest (e.g., patent, trademark, copyright, licensing agreement, etc.) in the Investigational Product being tested in the clinical study; and

❑ I have a significant equity interest (e.g., any ownership interest, stock option, or other financial interest, the value of which cannot be calculated with reference to publicly available prices) in (*insert sponsoring pharmaceutical company's name*).

This certification shall apply throughout the entire term of the clinical study and for one year following completion of the clinical study. If there is any change in the accuracy of the foregoing statements during such time period, I shall hereby agree that I will promptly notify (*insert sponsoring pharmaceutical company's name*).

_____

Signature of Principal Investigator   Date

*Tax ID#/Social Security # _____

Affiliated Institution _____

Tax ID# _____

Required for internal tracking only and will not be submitted to the FDA.

Form 15. Sample HIPAA Authorization to Access Protected Health Information

Protocol Title _____

Protocol # _____

Sponsor _____

Principal Investigator's Name _____

- ✔ Access to your Protected Health Information (PHI) will be required for the purpose of your participation in this research study.

- ✔ PHI is medical information that identifies you as an individual, such as name, address, social security number, and other personal details about you.

- ✔ This will include information that is used to determine your eligibility for the research study and is collected from the procedures that are carried out as part of the research study. This may include the following types of personal information:

    1. Your past medical history, including medical information from your primary care physician

    2. Physical exam, laboratory tests (blood and/or urine)

    3. Response to any study treatments you may receive

    4. Information related to study visits and phone calls

    5. Additional tests or procedures required by the Protocol

    6. Other information relating to your participation in this research study (include any study-specific information, i.e., x-ray, EKG, will need to be added here)

- ✔ With your permission, the Principal Investigator (study physician) and his/her research staff will be allowed to give this information to the research study Sponsor's key individuals. The Sponsor's key individuals include any person or company working for or with the Sponsor to facilitate the research study. They will have the right to see your health information and know your identity during and after research study.

- ✔ These key individuals agree to keep all of your information confidential, which will minimize the risk that it will be released to others without your permission.

- ✔ Permission to access your PHI will continue until such time as it is no longer required by the Sponsor of this research study.

- ✔ You have the right to see and copy any of the information gathered about you, but not until the research study is completed.

- ✔ You also have the right to withdraw this permission at any time by providing a *written request* to the research study physician. When you withdraw your permission, no new health information that might identify you will be gathered after that date, and you will not be able to continue participation in the research study. Information that has already been obtained may still be used by the Sponsor.

- ✔ By signing this authorization form, you are giving your permission to use and give out your PHI. If you do not give your permission, you will not be able to continue in this research study.

- ✔ You will be provided with a copy of this form for your personal files.

_____

Signature of Subject   Date

_____

Signature of Legally Authorized Representative (if applicable)   Date

_____

Authority of Subject's Personal Representative of Relationship to Subject
(when signed by a Legally Authorized Representative)

Form 16. STOP: Before Any Med Changes

STOP!

BEFORE ANY MED CHANGES
KINDLY CONTACT:

(INSERT NAME AND NUMBER OF PERSON RESPONSIBLE)

THIS PATIENT IS A PARTICIPANT
IN A RESEARCH PROJECT

Form 17. STOP: This Patient Is a Participant in a Research Project

STOP!

THIS PATIENT IS A PARTICIPANT IN A RESEARCH PROJECT

KINDLY CONTACT:
(INSERT NAME AND NUMBER OF PERSON RESPONSIBLE)

REGARDING THE FOLLOWING:

✔ PRIOR TO ANY CHANGES TO CURRENT MEDICATION

✔ <u>ANY</u> CHANGES IN THE PATIENT'S PHYSICAL CONDITION

✔ DATE AND TIME PATIENT WILL BE DISCHARGED

Form 18. Transporting Study Material from Main Site to Satellite Sites

Protocol Number: _____ Sponsor: _____

To Be Dispensed at Satellite Office

Site Location: _____

Principal Investigator: _____

Research Nurse: _____

Subject Initials: _____ Subject Number: _____

Lot Number: _____ Amount of Study Drug Sent: _____

Temperature at Packaging: _____ Time Sent: _____

Special Instructions: _____

_____

_____   _____

Signature of Person Transferring to Courier   Date

_____   _____

Signature of Research Nurse Receiving Study Drug   Date

SIGN AND FAX THIS FORM IMMEDIATELY UPON RECEIPT OF STUDY DRUG TO:

_____

Store Study Drug According to Instructions Noted on Form
Place Copy of This Form in Your Research Drug Accountability Log
RETURN OF UNUSED STUDY DRUG FROM SATELLITE OFFICE

_____   _____

Signature of Research Nurse Returning Unused Medication   Date

Amount Returned*: _____   Time Returned: _____

_____   _____

Signature of Research Nurse Returning Unused Mediation   Date

Amount Returned*: _____   Time Received: _____

*(*i.e., bottles; vials; blister packs*)

_____   _____

Signature of Research Nurse Verifying Return Study Drug Accountability   Date

Form 19. Sample Principal Investigator Delegation of Responsibility Form

PRINCIPAL INVESTIGATOR DELEGATION OF RESPONSIBILITIES

Sponsor: _____

Study Title: _____

Study #: _____

Principal Investigator: _____

Site Name: _____

Site Number: _____

List the names, signatures, initials and procedure responsibilities for those individuals participating in the conduct of this trial

Procedures Responsibilities Legend (For Reference Only)

1. Physical
2. History
3. Phlebotomy
4. Collecting Safety Data
5. Collecting Efficacy Data
6. Dispense Medication(s)
7. CRF Entry
8. Scheduling Study Visits
9. Performing Special Study Procedures

Name and Title *(please print)*	Listed on 1572?	Signature	Initials	Procedure Responsibilities *(Enter Applicable Number(s) from Above)*	Date(s)
Name: Title:	☐ No ☐ Yes				
Name: Title:	☐ No ☐ Yes				
Name: Title:	☐ No ☐ Yes				
Name: Title:	☐ No ☐ Yes				
Name: Title:	☐ No ☐ Yes				

Form 20. Sample Curriculum View Form

Name

Address (Use address of institution or where site research is being conducted)

Therapeutic Experience

Education

Professional Affiliations

Publications

Certifications:

Signature _____   Date _____

Suggestions:

- ✔ Try to use bullet points.
- ✔ Be brief; however, include pertinent information.

You do not have to note the following:

- ✔ Social security number
- ✔ Marital status
- ✔ Number of children
- ✔ Birth date

Form 21. Patient Assent Form

For patients seven and older

I have a disease called _____. This means I have _____.

I will be treated with _____. _____ may also be part of my treatment.

My doctor told me what this research study is about. I know this research is being done to learn more about _____ and how to treat it. There may be additional tests that will be done if I am part of this study.

I have been given time to think about being in this research study, and my questions have been answered. If I think of more questions later, I can call. Dr. _____ or ask next time I see Dr. _____.

I know I don't have to agree to be in this research study, and no one will be upset with me and I will still get treatment. It has been explained to me what treatment I will get if I decide not to be in this study.

Even though I agree now, I may feel differently later on. If I change my mind, it will be OK, and I will still be take care of by the doctors and nurses. I know that I may talk with my parents and/or doctors if I change my mind about being in the study at any time.

The doctors will tell me if they find out new things that they didn't know about when they first explained this study to me. Years from now when the study is all done, I will be able to find out from my doctor what was learned.

All the information collected about me for this study will be kept private, and my name will not be used on the study records. When the study is finished, the doctors will write a report about what was learned. This report will not include my name or that I was in the study.

If I sign my name at the end of this form, it means I agree to be in this study. I will be given a copy of this form to keep after I sign it and so will my parents.

Acknowledgment of Assent

_____

Printed Name of Participant (child is between 7 and 18 years of age)

_____

Signature of Participant

_____   _____
Investigator   Date   Signature of Person   Date
                                        Explaining Assent

Version Date:

_____
Witness Signature   Date

Waiver of Assent to Participate in a Clinical Research Project

Investigator Statement

Assent is waived because of the mental age, psychological state of the child, or because there is potential for medical benefit to the child by participating in this research protocol.

Acknowledgment of Waiver

_____   _____
Patient Signature   Date   Investigator   Date

_____   _____
Patient Signature   Date   Witness Signature   Date

_____
Signature of Person   Date
Explaining Assent

APPENDIX III: Conversion Tables

A. Conversion to Military Time

Military time is simple and logical. It is based on the fact that each day is composed of 24 hours numbered from 1 through 24. As with conventional time, the last two digits of military time are used to indicate the minute after the hour. For example, the conventional times 6:30 AM and 11:45 PM would be written in military times as 0630 and 2345, respectively.

1:00 AM = 0100	1:00 PM = 1300
2:00 AM = 0200	2:00 PM = 1400
3:00 AM = 0300	3:00 PM = 1500
4:00 AM = 0400	4:00 PM = 1600
5:00 AM = 0500	5:00 PM = 1700
6:00 AM = 0600	6:00 PM = 1800
7:00 AM = 0700	7:00 PM = 1900
8:00 AM = 0800	8:00 PM = 2000
9:00 AM = 0900	9:00 PM = 2100
10:00 AM = 1000	10:00 PM = 2200
11:00 AM = 1100	11:00 PM = 2300
12:00 PM = 1200	12:00 AM = 2400

IMPORTANT: Note that 12:00 midnight is written 2400 in military time. However, one never goes past 2400 hours. One minute past midnight becomes 0001, 30 minutes past midnight becomes 0030, etc., right up to 59 minutes past midnight, which is 0059. This time 1:00 AM then becomes 0100.

B. Measures and Equivalents

Volume

29.57 mL = 1 fluid ounce
473 mL = 1 pint
1 liter = 33.8 fluid ounces
3785 mL = 1 gallon
5 mL = 1 teaspoon
15 mL = 1 tablespoon or ½ fluid ounce

Weight

1 kilogram [kg] = 2.2 lbs
1 pound = 453.59 grams
1 ounce = 28.35 grams
1 gram = 15.432 grains
1 grain = 65 mg
1/2 grain = 32.4 mg
1/4 grain = 16.2 mg

Height

1 centimeter [cm] = 0.39 inches
1 inch = 2.54 cm
1 meter = 39.37 inches
1 micron = 1/1000 mm

Other useful measures

1 liter of water weighs 1 kg
1 mL of water weighs 1 gram

C. Conversion Charts for Height and Weight Measurements

Feet Inches	Inches	Centimeters
4' 8"	56	142.2
4' 9"	57	144.8
4' 10"	58	147.3
4' 11"	59	149.9
5' 0"	60	152.4
5' 1"	61	154.9
5' 2"	62	157.5
5' 3"	63	160.0
5' 4"	64	162.6
5' 5"	65	165.1
5' 6"	66	167.6
5' 7"	67	170.2
5' 8"	68	172.7
5' 9"	69	175.3
5' 10"	70	177.8
5' 11"	71	180.3
6' 0"	72	182.9
6' 1"	73	185.4
6' 2"	74	188.0
6' 3"	75	190.5
6' 4"	76	193.0
6' 5"	77	195.6
6' 6"	78	198.1
6' 7"	79	200.7
6' 8"	80	203.2

Pounds	Kilograms
1	0.4535
2.2046	1.0
95	43.1
100	45.4
105	47.6
110	49.9
115	52.2
120	54.4
125	56.7
130	59.0
135	61.2
140	63.5
145	65.8
150	68.0
155	70.3
160	72.6
165	74.8
170	77.1
175	79.4
180	81.6
185	83.9
190	86.2
195	88.5
200	90.7
205	93.0
210	95.3
215	97.5
220	99.8
225	102.1
230	104.3
235	106.6
240	108.9
245	111.1
250	113.4
255	115.7
260	117.9
265	120.2
270	122.5
275	124.7
280	127.0
285	129.3
290	131.5
295	133.8
300	136.1

APPENDIX IV: Common Terms and Acronyms

Acronym	Term
ADME	Absorption, Distribution, Metabolized, Excretion
ADR/AE	Adverse Drug Reaction/Adverse Event
CDA	Confidentiality Disclosure Agreement
CDM	Clinical Data Management
CFR	Code of Federal Regulations
CNS	Central Nervous System
CRA	Clinical Research Associate
CRO	Contract Research Organization
CRF	Case Report Form
CRS	Clinical Regulatory Specialist
DEA	Drug Enforcement Administration
EC	Ethics Committee
GCP	Good Clinical Practice
GLP	Good Laboratory Practice
HREC	Human Research Ethics Committees
HMO	Health Management Organization
IB	Investigator Brochure
IC	Informed Consent
ICF	Informed Consent Form
ICH	International Conference on Harmonisation
IEC	Independent Ethics Committee
IRB	Institutional Review Board
IRDB	Investigator Research Database
ISFN	Investigator Site File Notebook
LOI	Letter of Intent
LREC	Local Research Ethics Committee
MAP	Master Action Plan
MREC	Multi Research Ethics Committee (UK)
NDA	New Drug Application
PI	Principal Investigator
PIS	Patient Information Sheet
PM	Project Manager
PQRS	PPD Query Resolution System
QA	Quality Assurance
QC	Quality Control
RA	Research Assistant
RCM	Research Coordination Manager
RCR	Regulatory Compliance Review
RTMS	Research Trial Management System
SAE	Serious Adverse Event

SC	Study Coordinator
SMF	Study Master File
SMO	Site Management Organization
SOP	Standard Operating Procedures
TAL	Training Attendance Log
TMF	Trial Master File
WHO	World Health Organization

APPENDIX V: Glossary of Terms

Abbreviated New Drug Application (ANDA)
Simplified submission for products with the same or very closely related active ingredients, dosage form, use, strength, administration route, and labeling as a product that has already been shown to be safe and effective. An ANDA includes all the information on chemistry and manufacturing controls found in an NDA but does not usually have to include efficacy and safety data from studies in animals and humans. It must, however, contain evidence that the duplicate drug is bioequivalent to the previously approved drug.

Administrative Change
Change to a protocol involving only administrative details and having no impact on study design or subject safety. An administrative change requires IRB/IEC notification but does not require notification of regulatory agencies prior to implementation.

Adverse Event (AE)
Any untoward medical occurrence in a patient or clinical investigation subject administered a pharmaceutical product and that does not necessarily have a causal relationship with this treatment. An AE can therefore be any unfavorable and unintended sign (including an abnormal laboratory finding), symptom, or disease temporarily associated with the use of a medicinal (investigational) product, whether related to the medicinal (investigational) product or not. (See the ICH Guideline for Clinical Safety Data Management: Definitions and Standards for Expedited Reporting.) (ICH)

Altered Data
Generating biased data or changed data that is legitimately obtained. An example of an altered document includes unsupported changes to data on a document, such as exam dates, date of birth, etc. An example of altered data can include unsupported changes to data in the source document and/or the CRF.

Amended Protocol
A Protocol that has been revised or an amendment to the Protocol.

ANDA
Abbreviated New Drug Application.

ANDA Protocol Outline
Document that defines study design, reference formulation, and basic pharmacokinetics of compound to be tested.

Application
A formal request for review and approval, where issue of an opinion/approval by the regulatory authority is required for the trial commencement.

Archival	The process of performing a full backup of a project's study data, meta-data, and associated files to tape for long-term storage at an offsite facility.
ARSAC	Administration of Radioactive Substances Advisory Committee.
Audit	A systematic and independent examination of trial-related activities and documents to determine whether the evaluated trial-related activities were conducted, and whether the data was recorded, analyzed, and accurately reported according to the Protocol, Sponsor's SOPs, GCP, and the applicable regulatory requirement(s). (ICH GCP 1.6)
Audit-Related Documents	Written evaluations by a regulatory agency or a quality assurance group (internal or external) that contain findings and observations about PPD activities.
Author	Person writing any section of the Investigator Brochure. May be a member of the medical writing, clinical pharmacology, medical affairs, or regulatory affairs staff.
Becquerel	(Bq) Radiological unit, source strength.
Bind	To place yourself under legal obligation and/or to cause you to be legally responsible.
Blinding/Masking	A procedure in which one or more parties to the trial are kept unaware of the treatment assignment(s). Single-blinding usually refers to the subject(s) being unaware, and double-blinding usually refers to the subject(s), investigator(s), monitor, and, in some cases, data analyst(s) being unaware of the treatment assignment(s). (ICH)
Blood	Means human blood, human blood components, and products made from human blood.
Bloodborne Pathogens	Means pathogenic microorganisms that are present in human blood and can cause disease in humans. These pathogens include, but are not limited to, HBV virus (HBV) and human immunodeficiency virus (HIV).

BMI (Body Mass Index)	This is a value obtained when weight is divided by height. The formula used for calculation of this value is BMI = Weight (Kg) / Height (m) x Height (m).
Call Center Services (CCS)	The area where the telephone operators use computers and telephone equipment to assist in subject/site recruitment and/or site support programs.
Call Center Services Questionnaire	The combined document of standardized opening remarks relative to the nature of clinical research, research subject rights, and confidentiality along with standardized study specific questions used to collect data from potential subjects; sometimes referred to as "script" or "transcript."
Call Center Services Site	Participating institutions or clinics that have provided documentation of respective advertisement approval, as needed, and that are Sponsor- or Clincal Operations-approved recipients of CCS efforts.
Call Center Services Staff (Operators)	Personnel who receive and record information by telephone from prospective study subjects and/or consumers pursuant to CCS advertising and recruitment programs.
Call Report	For purposes of this procedure, record of a specific Technical Support Communication. Use of the word "call" does not imply that these reports originate exclusively from telephone contact.
Case Report Form (CRF)	A printed, optical, or electronic document designed to record all of the Protocol-required information to be reported to the sponsor on each trial subject. (ICH)
Casebook Guide	Instructions for completing the CRF that may include sample completed CRF pages.
Causality	Relationship of an investigational product to an AE. Many causality categories are used to describe the degree of attributability of a product to an AE, such as Definite, Probable, Possible, Remote, Not Related; however, currently, there is no standard nomenclature.
Central Laboratory	Primary laboratory used by all investigators participating in a study for the analysis of specimens (e.g., biological fluids and tissue).

Centralized Recruitment Program A specific recruitment campaign consisting of one or more advertising media and support materials directed to either potential research subjects or consumers.

Certified Copy An exact copy of the original with initial and date of individual making the copy from the original with a statement that this is a true exact copy.

CFR Code of Federal Regulations.

Clinical Data Management Department responsible for managing database generation through data entry, data review, and data clean-up using data collected from a clinical study.

Clinical Monitor The person responsible for monitoring the conduct and progress of the clinical trial.

Clinical Research Associate (CRA) Appropriately trained sponsor representative or contracted individual who is responsible for overseeing the conduct of a clinical study. The CRA makes periodic visits to the trial site before, during, and at the conclusion of a study, to ascertain that the clinical Protocol is being adhered to and that all aspects of GCP are followed. Also synonymous with monitor.

Clinical Trial Materials Articles used in the conduct of a clinical trial, excluding investigational product. (Examples of clinical trial materials include CRFs, patient diaries, laboratory kits, thermometers.)

Clinical Trial/Study Any investigation in human subjects intended to discover or verify the clinical, pharmacological, and/or other pharmacodynamic effects of an investigational product(s), and/or to identify any adverse reactions to an investigational product(s), and/or to study absorption, distribution, metabolism, and excretion of an investigational product(s) with the object of ascertaining its safety and/or efficacy. The terms "clinical trial" and "clinical study" are synonymous. (ICH)

Clinical Trial/Study Report A written description of a trial/study of any therapeutic, prophylactic, or diagnostic agent conducted in human subjects, in which the clinical and statistical description, presentations, and analyses are fully integrated into a single report. (See the ICH Guideline for Structure and Content of Clinical Study Reports.)

Clintrial Database Administrator	The individual who provides user support and administration, security, and other operational support for Clintrial database activities.
Co-investigators	Investigators having equal power and responsibilities for a clinical trial.
Communications	Communications include written, verbal, or electronic communication such as, but not limited to, letters, memoranda, facsimile transmissions, electronic mail messages, voice mail messages, telephone conversations, and meetings.
Compassionate Use	Sometimes used to describe a request by a practitioner to treat a single patient with an investigational product. The request is usually in response to a desperate situation, such as the lack of approved or generally recognized treatments or the patient being unresponsive to other therapies.
Computer System Validation	Documented evidence, to a high degree of assurance, that the computer system performs its intended functions accurately and reliably.
Confidentiality	Prevention of disclosure, to other than authorized individuals, and/or Sponsor's propriety information or of a subject's identity. (ICH derived)
Confidentiality Agreement	Document preventing disclosure of facts to third parties. Also synonymous with Secrecy Agreement.
Contact Report	Written record of contact between a Sponsor's employee and trial site staff, client company, contract service agency, or regulatory agency.
Contaminated Laundry	Laundry that has been soiled with blood, body fluids, or other potentially infectious materials.
Contaminated Sharps	Any contaminated object that can penetrate the skin including, but not limited to, needles, scalpels, broken glass, broken capillary tubes, and exposed ends of dental wires.
Contamination	The presence or the reasonably anticipated presence of blood or other potentially infectious materials on an item or surface.
Contract Research Organization (CRO)	A person or an organization (commercial, academic, or other) contracted by the sponsor to perform one or more of a Sponsor's trial-related duties and functions. (ICH GCP 1.20)

Debarment	The FDA, authorized by the U.S. Generic Drug Enforcement Act (1992), has the right to forbid or deny individuals and/or firms from participation in the development of an investigational product. Those individuals/firms having been debarred are published in the U.S. Federal Register.
Declaration of Helsinki	International document defining the ethical principles under which clinical research is to be conducted.
Decontamination	The use of physical or chemical means to remove, inactivate, and destroy bloodborne pathogens. Pathogens must be destroyed on a surface or item to the point where they are no longer capable of transmitting infectious particles and the surface or item is rendered safe for handling, use, or disposal.
Deliverable	Any report text, table, listing, and figure or database produced for delivery to the client.
Designee	Individual empowered to sign agreements or perform actions through their position in an organization.
Dispensing Investigational Product	The act of providing investigational product to a subject wherein the study personnel inject, apply, or observe the physical administration of investigational product on or by the subject.
Dosing	The act of providing a unit dose or applying an investigational product to a subject wherein the study personnel inject, apply, or observe the physical administration of the investigational product on or by the subject.
Dosing Error	When an incorrect dose of investigational product has been inadvertently given to a subject, or taken by a subject, including dispensing or administering to the wrong subject or taking/administering the study medication on the wrong day or time, having taken/administered the wrong investigational product.
Drug Enforcement Administration (DEA)	Lead agency in the U.S. responsible for enforcing the controlled substance laws and regulations of the U.S.
Exposure Incident	A specific eye, mouth, other mucous membrane, nonintact skin, or parenteral contact with blood or other potentially infectious materials that result from the performance of an employee's duties.
FDA	Food and Drug Administration.

Financial Agreement	Document containing details of all financial arrangements entered into between the client company and/or a trial site. The financial agreement may form part of the Study Site Agreement (e.g., Statement of Agreement).
Fraud	Deliberate reporting of false or misleading data or the withholding of reportable data. Fraud does not include the submitting of poor quality data without the intent to deceive.
Good Clinical Practice (GCP)	A standard for the design, conduct, performance, monitoring, auditing, recording, analyses, and reporting of clinical trials that provides assurance that the data and reported results are credible and accurate, and that the rights, integrity, and confidentiality of trial subjects are protected. (ICH)
Hand-Washing Facilities	A facility providing an adequate supply of running potable water, soap, and single-use towels or hot air drying machines.
HAV	Hepatitis A Virus.
HBV	Hepatitis B Virus.
HCV	Hepatitis C Virus
HIV	Human Immunodeficiency Virus, the causative agent in Acquired Immune Deficiency Syndrome (AIDS).
ICH	International Conference on the Harmonization of Technical Requirements for registration of Pharmaceuticals for Human Use—a group of worldwide regulatory agencies and professional trade organizations formed to provide global standards for pharmaceutical development in the U.S., Europe, and Japan.
IND	Investigational New Drug Application.
IND Study	Study conducted in accordance with the requirements of the FDA Investigational New Drug regulations.
Indemnification	Process to relieve the investigator, subinvestigators, IRB/IEC, and/or research institution of responsibility against hurt, loss, or damage to subjects resulting from participation in a clinical trial.
Independent Ethics Committee (IEC)	An independent body (a review board or a committee, institutional, regional, national, or supranational), constituted of medical/scientific professionals and nonmedical/nonscientific members,

whose responsibility it is to ensure the protection of the rights, safety, and well-being of human subjects involved in a trial and to provide public assurance of that protection, by, among other things, reviewing and approving/providing favorable opinion on the trial protocol, the suitability of the investigator(s), facilities, and the methods and material to be used in obtaining and documenting informed consent of the trial subjects. The legal status, composition, function, operations, and regulatory requirements pertaining to Independent Ethics Committees may differ among countries, but should allow the Independent Ethics Committee to act in agreement with GCP as described in this guideline. (ICH)

Informational Translation — Informational translations are used where the original document remains the reference document, but translations of all or part of it will assist other parties in the review of documents. Examples are the translation of all or part of the local Investigational Ethics Committee approval letter or an Investigator CV.

Informed Consent — A process by which a subject voluntarily confirms his or her willingness to participate in a particular trial, after having been informed of all aspects of the trial that are relevant to the subject's decision to participate. Informed consent is documented by means of a written, signed, and dated informed consent form. (ICH)

Informed Consent Document — Document prepared in nontechnical language to provide clinical trial subjects with information detailing trial procedures, potential benefits, risks and inconveniences, and the subject's rights. This document is used to obtain proof of the subject's agreement to enter a study.

Inspection — The act by a regulatory authority(ies) of conducting an official review of documents, facilities, records, and any other resources that are deemed by the authority(ies) to be related to the clinical trial and that may be located at the site of the trial, at the sponsor's and/or contract research organization's (CRO) facilities, or at other establishments deemed appropriate by the regulatory authority(ies). (ICH GCP 1.29)

Installation Qualification (IQ) — Documented evidence that installation instructions were followed for computer system hardware and/or software.

Institutional Review Board (IRB) — An independent body constituted of medical, scientific, and nonscientific members, whose responsibility it is to ensure the protection of the rights, safety, and well-being of human subjects involved in a trial by, among other things, reviewing, approving, and providing continuing review of trials, of protocols and amendments, and of the methods and material to be used in obtaining and documenting informed consent of the trial subjects. (ICH)

Interactive Voice Response System (IVRS)

Automated central randomization system allowing investigators to obtain subject randomization information by telephone by use of interactive voice technology or a touch-tone keypad. IVRS systems may also control distribution of investigational product to sites.

International Conference on Harmonisation (ICH)

Group of worldwide regulatory agencies and professional trade organizations formed to provide harmonization of technical requirements for the development of pharmaceutical products.

Investigational New Drug Application (IND)

The application for an exemption from the U.S. Federal law requiring an approved NDA prior to shipping a drug in interstate commerce. The IND contains the clinical development plan for the drug, including as complete a picture as possible of the compound (e.g., structural formula), chemistry and manufacturing information, and the results of animal pharmacology and toxicology studies with the drug.

Investigational Product

A pharmaceutical form of an active ingredient or placebo being tested or used as a reference in a clinical trial, including a product with a market authorization when used or assembled (formulated or packaged) in a way different from the approved form, or when used for an unapproved indication, or when used to gain further information about an approved use. (ICH)

Investigational Product Labels

Labels attached to inner and outer containers of investigational products containing all information sufficient to identify the product and meet local regulations for such products.

Investigational Product Release

Regulatory compliance personnel's authorization to ship investigational product.

Investigator

One or more persons responsible for the practical performance of a clinical trial and for the integrity, health, and welfare of the subjects during the trial. The investigator is an appropriately qualified, trained, and experienced person, particularly in the clinical area of the proposed trial, who is familiar with the background and the requirements of the study. If a trial is conducted by a team of individuals at a trial site, the investigator is the responsible leader of the team and may be called the principal investigator.

Investigator Meeting	Meeting to provide training to investigators and other trial site staff on all aspects of a clinical study.
Investigator Site File	File that is prepared for or by the investigator prior to study initiation and contains copies of documents relating to the clinical study. It is kept at the trial site, updated by the investigator and reviewed by the monitor at the monitoring visits. It must be retained by the investigator for a fixed period after the study is completed. Also known as Site Regulatory Binder or Regulatory Binder.
Investigator's Brochure	A compilation of the clinical and nonclinical data on the investigational product(s) that is relevant to the study of the investigational product(s) in human subjects. The information must be updated during the course of the clinical program, as new data are generated. (ICH derived)
IRMER	Ionising Radiation (Medical Exposure) Regulations (2000).
Laboratory	A workplace where diagnostic or other screening procedures are performed on blood or other potentially infectious materials.
Licensed Healthcare Professional	A person whose legally permitted scope of practice allows him or her to independently perform the activities required.
Manufactured or Fabricated Data	Data or information created without performing the tasks required to get the data. This includes data that is not supported by the presence of reasonably expected source documentation. An example of a fabricated document includes a document that has been created and submitted for a particular study subject, but that does not actually belong to that subject and lacks source documentation for items such as lab findings, chest x-rays, and concomitant medications.
Meaningful Pain Relief	The time point at which the patient feels that they have had a significant amount of pain relief post dose.
Monitor	See Clinical Research Associate.
Monitoring	The act of overseeing the progress of a clinical trial, and of ensuring that it is conducted, recorded, and reported in accordance with the Protocol, SOPs, GCP, and the applicable regulatory requirement(s). (ICH)

Multicenter Trial/Study	A clinical trial conducted according to a single Protocol but at more than one site, and, therefore, carried out by more than one investigator. (ICH)
NDA	New Drug Application.
Needleless Systems	Devices that do not use needles for administration of medication or fluids or collection of blood or body fluids after initial access is established.
New Drug Application (NDA)	Application requesting FDA approval to market a new drug for human use.
Notification	Notification is the act of giving notice or information to the regulatory authority, but where review of documents or issue of an opinion/approval by the authority is not required for trial commencement (an acknowledgment of receipt may be provided).
Obligations	Responsibilities for aspects of the control, management, and conduct of a clinical trial.
Occupational Exposure	Reasonably anticipated skin, eye, mucous membrane, or parenteral contact with blood or other potentially infectious materials that may result from the performance of an employee's duties.
Omitted Data	Data that has an impact on the study outcome and is not reported to the CRF. An example of omitted data includes the failure to correctly report exclusion criteria.
Pain Relief Scale	A categorical scale (none, a little, some, a lot, complete) for indicating the level of pain relief being experienced by a patient.
Pain Scale	A categorical scale (none, mild, moderate, severe) for indicating the level of pain being experienced by a patient.
Perceptible Pain Relief	The time point at which the patient feels that they first perceive pain relief post dose.
Potential Investigator	Individual who is being considered to conduct a clinical trial.
Potentially Infectious Material	Blood or body fluid that may potentially contain a bloodborne pathogen, such as blood or semen, vaginal secretions, cerebrospinal

fluid, synovial fluid, pleural fluid, peritoneal fluid, amniotic fluid, or pericardial fluid. Saliva or any body fluid or tissue where it is difficult or impossible to determine contamination must also be considered infectious.

Procedural Documents   Standard Operating Procedures.

Program   Any activity associated with a Protocol, consisting of advertising media and/or support materials directed to potential research subjects, CCS sites, or consumers.

Program Files   Consist of documents pertaining to the conduct of a CCS program, including, but not limited to final IRB/IEC approved Protocol/advertisements, final approved screening questionnaires, internal/external communication and CCS training/QA documentation, and are stored in the CCS file room and serve as an archive for all program-specific information.

Program Manager   Individual who directs a drug development program that may include many separate projects.

Project   The evaluation of a company or other entity for potential merger, acquisition, strategic joint venture, or other similar form of collaboration.

Project Manager   Individual functionally responsible for the coordination and management of activities associated with all or part of a project.

Project-Specific Documents   Extensive working instructions or comprehensive procedures applicable to certain projects, tasks, or locations.

Project Team   Assigned representatives from each functional group involved in performing the project workscope (e.g., Biostatistics, Data Management, Clinical, PVG, Regulatory, and Medical Writing).

Proprietary   Information or product that is owned by an individual or company that may be protected under a copyright or patent. Such information is considered to be a trade secret and is not to be disseminated without the written consent of the individual or company.

Protocol	A document that describes the objective(s), design, methodology, statistical considerations, and organization of a trial. The Protocol usually also gives the background and rationale for the trial, but these could be provided in other Protocol referenced documents. Throughout the ICH/GCP guidelines, the term Protocol refers to Protocol and Protocol amendments. (ICH)
Protocol Amendment	Change to a clinical Protocol that affects the safety of subjects, the scope of the investigation, or the scientific quality of the study. Requires IRB/IEC approval, and notification and/or approval of regulatory agencies prior to implementation.
Protocol Author	Individual responsible for coordinating development of a clinical Protocol.
Protocol Number	Unique identifying code for a clinical Protocol.
Protocol Violation	Failure to comply with the Protocol that results in a significant added risk to the subject; failure by the subject or investigator to adhere to significant (inclusion/exclusion/primary endpoint criteria defined by the clinical team) Protocol requirements yet the subject is enrolled and/or continuing in the study without prior client company approval; and noncompliance to GCP (FDA regulations and/or ICH GCP guidelines).
Quality Assurance	All those planned and systematic actions that are established to ensure that the trial is performed and the data are generated, documented (recorded), and reported in compliance with GCP and applicable regulatory requirements. (ICH)
Quality Control	The operational techniques and activities undertaken to verify that the requirements for quality of the trial-related activities have been fulfilled. (ICH derived)
Query	Request for the clarification of an item contained in a CRF (e.g., clarification of inaccuracy, discrepancy, or item requiring resolution).
Randomization	The process of assigning trial subjects to treatment or control groups using an element of chance to determine the assignments in order to reduce bias. (ICH)

Randomization Code	A schedule identifying the treatment each subject will receive during each study period while participating in a clinical trial.
Randomization Team	Individuals involved in the generation, receipt, storage, or distribution of randomization information. It must include at least one degreed statistician and at least one quality reviewer. Each team member must have a designated and comparably qualified backup. Randomization team members must not serve as project team members on any project where they also function as randomization team members.
Regulatory Agency Report	Notification of facts to a regulatory agency, which may be made periodically (e.g., annual updates) or as required (e.g., serious adverse event reporting).
Regulatory Authority	National body (e.g., Food and Drug Administration [FDA]; Medicines Control Agency [MCA]; Bundesinstitut für Arzneimittel und Medizinprodukte [BfArM]; Health Protection Branch [HPB], etc.) controlling the use and approval of medicinal products and devices.
Rescue Medication	The pain relief medication provided to the patient at their request if the patient does not achieve adequate pain relief from the study medication.
Research Agreement	Shall mean any agreement entered into between CRO/SMO or the client company and the investigator regarding a particular study. The Research Agreement shall set forth all obligations and services to be performed by the investigator in compensation therefore.
RPA	Radiation Protection Advisor.
RPS	Radiation Protection Supervisor.
Safety Monitor	Person responsible for the review and evaluation of information relevant to the safety of the drug (listed on Line 15 of the Form FDA 1571).
Safety Physician/Medical Monitor	A physician designated to be responsible for monitoring medical safety of the subjects in a given study, including, but not limited to, unblinding, AE reporting, and management.

Senior Statistical Reviewer	A senior statistician who performs experimental statistical review to ensure scientific integrity of all Biostatistics deliverables and the Study Report, as assigned by Biostatistics Management.
Serious Adverse Event/Experience (SAE) or Serious Adverse Drug Reaction (Serious ADR)	Any adverse drug experience occurring at any dose that results in any of the following outcomes: • death • life-threatening, that is, any event that (in the opinion of the Investigator) poses an immediate risk of death from that event • inpatient hospitalization • prolongation of existing hospitalization • persistent or significant disability/incapacity • congenital anomaly/birth defect Important medical events that may not result in death, be life-threatening, or require hospitalization may be considered a serious adverse drug experience when, based upon appropriate medical judgment, they may jeopardize the patient or subject and may require medical or surgical intervention.
Significant Communication	Any information that, in the opinion of the project team, may potentially affect the conduct of the study.
Site Assessment	Procedure to check that a trial site has the appropriate facilities, staff, and subject population to conduct a study in accordance with the Protocol and GCP. Also synonymous with Prestudy Assessment.
Site Close-out	Process of completing a clinical study at a trial site. Site close-out may start when the last subject has completed treatment/follow-up, but is not complete until all data queries relating to the site have been resolved.
Site Initiation	Procedures surrounding the start of a clinical study at a trial site (e.g., checking site facilities, delivery of clinical supplies, etc.). Unless waived by the client company, usually an initiation visit will be performed before any subjects are entered into a clinical study.
Site Visit Log	Document maintained at the trial site that records visits to the site by Sponsor representatives.
Source Data	All information in original records and certified copies of original records of clinical findings, observations, or other activities in a clinical trial necessary for the reconstruction and evaluation of the trial.

Source data are contained in source documents (original records or certified copies).

Source Document Original documents, data, and records (e.g., hospital records, clinical and office charts, laboratory notes, memoranda, subjects' diaries or evaluation checklists, pharmacy dispensing records, recorded data from automated instruments, copies or transcriptions certified after verification as being accurate and complete, microfiches, photographic negatives, microfilm or magnetic media, x-rays, subject files, and records kept at the pharmacy, at the laboratories, and at medico-technical departments involved in the clinical trial). (ICH)

Source Document Verification Visual check of the data presented in a CRF against source documents to ensure that the source data exist and have been transcribed accurately.

Sponsor An individual company, institution, or organization that takes responsibility for the initiation, management, and/or financing of a clinical trial. (ICH GCP 1.53)

Standard Operating Procedure (SOP) The detailed written instructions to achieve uniformity of the performance of a specific function. (ICH GCP 1.55)

Statistical Reviewer Person who reviews the statistical aspects of the report. Should include product statistician and, as appropriate, Senior Biostatistician.

Study Coordinator Person who generally handles the administrative responsibilities of a clinical trial at the site and acts as a liaison between the trial site and PPD.

Study Discontinuation Premature closure of a trial site for operational reasons (e.g., poor recruitment, poor compliance), other reasons connected with the conduct of the study, or a change to the clinical development strategy.

Study Documentation All documents supplied by an investigator or obtained by a client company that are required to ensure a site has been set up in accordance with GCP requirements.

Study Master File Files containing documents and records (electronic or hard-copy) related to the general nature of the study, its development, and conduct.

Study Site Agreement	Documentation signed by the investigator or authorized person containing details of the work to be done, responsibilities of the investigator and client company, and general conduct of the study. Also synonymous with Statement of Agreement (SOA).
Study Supplies	Materials used in a study, including the investigational product(s).
Subinvestigator	Any individual member of the clinical trial team designated and supervised by the investigator at a trial site to perform critical trial-related procedures and/or to make important trial-related decisions (e.g., associates, residents, research fellows). (ICH)
Subject Identification List	Confidential list maintained by the trial site containing adequate information to uniquely identify a subject.
Subject/Trial Subject	An individual who participates in a clinical trial, either as a recipient of the investigational product(s) or as a control. (ICH)
Tape	The term tape is used to refer to magnetic tape but could refer to other backup media such as CD-ROM.
Trefoil	Radioactive warning sign.
Trial Site	The location(s) where trial-related activities are actually conducted. (ICH)
Unexpected Adverse Event	Any AE that is not identified in nature, severity, or frequency in the current labeling or investigator's brochure, or that is not described in the risk information in the investigator's brochure, Protocol, or general study plan.
Universal Precautions	Treating all human body fluids, specimens, and items contaminated with blood or body fluids as potentially infectious. Such material may contain bloodborne pathogens.
Validation	The process of independently verifying the accuracy and completeness of the programming related to Biostatistics and Data Management deliverables.
Validation Program	A program written to verify that a production program functions correctly.

Validator   The Biostatistics team member(s) assigned to validate the Biostatistics and Data Management deliverables.

Visual Analog Scale   A 100 mm line scale for indicating the level of pain being experienced by a patient, i.e., no pain to worst pain.

Whole Document   A whole document translation may be required for documents that
Translation   will become a reference document at a study site. Examples are the translation of a Protocol, study subject diary cards, investigator's brochure, informed consent, etc.

About the Author

Deborrah Norris* has worked in the pharmaceutical industry for more than 20 years. She started in the industry as a Clinical Research Coordinator, has worked as a Clinical Research Associate, CRA Manager, and Project Manager and Director for several major pharmaceutical companies, and is certified to conduct site audits of clinical trials.

She has a wide range of experience in many therapeutic areas, and Ms. Norris has made significant contributions to the development of new compounds. Her experience in the industry includes, but is not limited to, medical writing and the training of allied health professionals on the clinical development process and GCP/ICH guidelines.

Ms. Norris has presented at several international conferences and has performed training for European Clinical Research Associates for several major pharmaceutical companies, including the development of videotaped material used as an adjunct to the presented training materials. She has also been invited to present internationally on pertinent informed consent issues.

Ms. Norris's *Clinical Research Coordinator Handbook* was the first handbook published to provide Clinical Research Coordinators with information to assist them in their role as a Study Coordinator. She has written four editions of this handbook, one of which was translated and published in Japan. The Third Edition received a favorable review from the *Good Clinical Practices Journal*. In addition, her publications are used to teach both GCP/ICH guidelines in several medical schools across the country. She also authored the book, *Glossary of Lay Language Synonyms for Common Terms Used in Informed Consent Documents for Clinical Studies: A Handbook for Clinical Researchers* (Information Today, Inc., 1996).

Ms. Norris prides herself on her ethics and ability to work successfully with Study Coordinators to ensure the successful completion of clinical trials. As a former Clinical Research Coordinator, she recognizes the valuable role of a Study Coordinator to the success of any clinical trial. She believes the Study Coordinator is the heart of research.

*Deborrah Norris is the pen name used for her publications to avoid any perception of utilizing her site relationships to purchase her publications in order to obtain financial gain.